INTEGRATED MEDICINE FOR NEUROLOGIC DISORDERS

Herbs and Nutrients for Alzheimer's Disease, Parkinson's Disease, Multiple Sclerosis, Stroke, Migraine, and Seizures

SIDNEY KURN, M.D.

SHERYL SHOOK, Ph.D.

Health Press NA Inc.
Albuquerque, New Mexico

Published by Health Press NA Inc.
Albuquerque, NM 87176

Library of Congress Cataloging in Publication Data
Kurn, Sidney, 1943-
Integrated medicine for neurologic disorders : herbs and nutrients for Alzheimer's disease, Parkinson's disease, multiple sclerosis, stroke, migraine, and seizures / Sidney Kurn, Sheryl Shook.
        p. ; cm.
Includes bibliographical references and index.
                        ISBN-13: 978-0-929173-50-4
1. Herbs--Therapeutic use. 2. Dietary supplements. 3. Nervous system--Diseases--Diet therapy. 4. Nervous system--Diseases--Alternative treatment. 5. Integrative medicine. I. Shook, Sheryl, 1963- II. Title.
    [DNLM: 1. Nervous System Diseases--diet therapy. 2. Dietary Supplements. 3. Holistic Health. 4. Nervous System Diseases--drug therapy. 5. Phytotherapy. WL 140 K96i 2007]
RC350.H47K87 2007
616.8'04654--dc22   2007033662
ISBN: 978-0-929173-50-4
Cover Design by Florence J. Plecki

Disclaimer: *Integrated Medicine for Neurologic Disorders* is a presentation of the empirical basis for the use of herbs and nutrients in various neurologic disorders. The information presented in this book has been obtained from authentic and reliable sources. Although great care has been taken to ensure the accuracy of the information presented, the authors and the publisher cannot assume responsibility for the validity of all materials or the consequences for their use. Before starting any regimen of vitamins, supplements, or herbs, you should consult with your physician.

The editors have made every effort to identify trademarked products within the text of the book accurately; however, it is impossible to check each instance.

Acknowledgments

This is the sweetest part of writing a book, repaying in small measure the debt an author owes with thanks and gratitude. My biggest creditor is Vicki, my wife, who suffered my hours of oblivious distraction as I summoned my concentration on this book. Her support, confidence and affection created the momentum to bring the book to fruition. Second is my co-author Sheryl – who patiently turned my Zen brush strokes into real substance. The readable, detailed form of the book belongs to her. Without the belief and assiduous efforts of her husband, Doug, this book would never have found itself in print. Thanks to the many patients who have taught me so much for so long and for whom this book was actually written. Thanks to the staff of Farmacopia over the last 11 years. They are the really "green" people who have softened the edges of my medical training and taught me some of the real mysteries of herbs, nutrients and healing. And to two of my formal teachers, Lois Johnson, M.D., and David Hoffmann who helped guide me into the greener world of real medicine. And finally, to many friends over the years, including Wayne Souza Pharm. D., L. Ac. who answered my queries and taught me by example, and who keep alive the deep humanism so important in the healing arts.

Sidney Kurn, M.D.

As I reflect upon the compassionate individuals that have shared my journey, I am filled with appreciation for their unwavering support. My deepest gratitude goes to my loving and kind husband, Doug Fetterly, who continually inspires me with his graciousness and wisdom. The time we spend, side-by-side, writing our own books and editing each other's manuscripts, is the sweetest part of my work. With her lyrical spirit and thoughtfulness, my daughter, Mary, continues to provide me with abundant joy and love. She showed endless patience throughout her childhood as she accompanied me to work in the lab, hospital, and classroom. Without Sid, my co-author, this book would not have been possible. He warmly welcomed me into this project and gave me the pleasure of a respectful and purely positive collaboration. I am grateful to my dear friend, Debbie Zakerski, who came into my life and taught me, and continues to remind me, what really matters. I am thankful for my parents, Sherry and Coy Shook, who encouraged me throughout my pursuits and filled my life with goodness and love. Kami McBride facilitated the big beautiful step I took into the world of herbal healing. Thanks to Lois Johnson, M.D., for bringing Sid and me together. I would like to thank Kathleen Frazier and Florence Plecki, at Health Press for putting our book into the hands of others.

Sheryl Shook, Ph.D.

Dedication

Integrated Medicine for Neurologic Disorders is dedicated to thousands of patients over the last thirty years. Instead of cursing the darkness, they light a candle to find undiscovered truths. Faced by daunting and, at times, unrelenting suffering from neurologic illness, their collective courage has widened the boundaries of standard therapies for their disorders. This book is a small offering of our gratitude for their priceless gift of sharing their path of discovery with us.

May we strive for "science with humanity" as advised by Mahatma Gandhi.

Contents

Preface

Integrated Medicine for Neurologic Disorders was initially compiled from lectures and handouts, introducing practitioners, patients, and their families to the judicious use of supplements in various neurologic disorders. Each chapter arose in slightly different contexts and varied in terms of description of the disorder, the relationship of herbs and nutrients to the underlying disease mechanisms, and a practical summary at the end. Rather than edit the chapters to fit one template, the authors and publisher decided to preserve the original uniqueness of each chapter. This variety of format reflects the enthusiasm of the authors for certain topics, particularly regarding disease mechanisms, prompted by new discoveries in neurologic science. These discoveries, although introduced and discussed in one chapter, could appear in different chapters. For example, the proteasome, protein homeostasis, and resveratrol appear in the chapter about Parkinson's disease but easily could have been introduced in the Alzheimer's disease chapter. The summaries and charts at the ends of each chapter are designed for accessibility and practicality. As a reference, the reader could start with the summary first, before reading the body of the chapter. This book is dedicated to all the patients who have suffered from these disorders, and taught the authors so much over their professional careers. We hope this book helps relieve some of this suffering.

Introduction

Integrated Medicine for Neurologic Disorders is offered to the reader as a practical and in-depth approach to the use of supplements in six neurologic conditions: multiple sclerosis (MS), Parkinson's disease (PD), stroke, Alzheimer's disease (AD), migraine, and epilepsy. It draws from the extended clinical experience of one author in combining standardized and alternative approaches in clinical practice and from the neuroscience scholarship and insight of the other author. Although standard pharmaceutical approaches have much to offer, most neurologic patients, as well as their treating neurologists, will attest to their limitations. This is particularly true in the neurodegenerative disorders. The prevention of recurrent stroke may be more amenable to standard treatment through the treatment of risk factors for atherosclerosis (hardening of the arteries).

Scientific research has begun to uncover the existence of a few abnormal processes, such as inflammation, which may be found in four of the disorders discussed in this book (PD, AD, MS and stroke). For example, MS has long been known to be an inflammatory disorder involving the myelin or white matter of the brain. More recently, an inflammatory component has been demonstrated in the other three disorders, including the atherosclerotic plaques of blood vessels that can break apart, moving downstream to deprive the brain of its vital nutrient, oxygen. This is a common cause of stroke. Although the nature of the inflammation may differ somewhat from one disorder to the next, it is inflammation, nonetheless. This offers hope that an anti-inflammatory drug used in arthritis, for example, may have a practical application in these disorders as well. Even the common drug ibuprofen may have an application in AD.[1] This suggests that certain herbs or nutrients, known to have anti-inflammatory properties, may also be useful for reducing the inflammatory component of these diseases. Turmeric, for example, has multiple upstream and downstream anti-inflammatory effects including interference with the intracellular transcription molecule NF-kappa B, the pervasive pro-inflammatory signaling molecule, tumor necrosis factor (TNF), and a number of enzymes and other substances at the site of inflammation itself including phospholipase, lipooxygenase, Cyclooxygenase-2, matrix metalloproteinases, and nitric oxide.[2,3,4] Another potent antioxidant with multiple sites of action is N-acetyl cysteine (NAC). Derived from the sulfur-containing amino acid cysteine, NAC stimulates the intracellular production of glutathione (GSH), a potent, essential antioxidant that is poorly absorbed when taken by mouth. Similar to turmeric, NAC has several upstream anti-inflammatory effects including the reduction of TNF and NF-kappa B levels.

The oxidative theory of aging and disease dates back at least to 1954 with the work of Denham Harmon M.D., Ph.D. While working at Berkeley's Donner Laboratory, Dr. Harmon, after years of reflection, had the epiphany that free radical reactions, or oxidation, so pervasive in biochemistry, could explain the universal aging of biological systems. Subsequent research has shown a direct relationship between free radical damage and disorders as diverse as cataracts, wrinkling of skin, cancer, and the neurodegenerative disorders, particularly PD. Recent research documents a key role of oxidative stress in MS,[5] AD,[6] and atherosclerosis.[7]

Although the mechanism of oxidative stress may differ from one disorder to another, nutrients and herbs offer a large variety of antioxidants to quench the limited number of free radicals involved in these disorders. Basic and clinical research supports the use of the more common antioxidants such as vitamins C and E, alpha-lipoic acid (ALA), and as many different flavonoids found in fruits, vegetables, and herbs. The human antioxidant system involves multiple components that interact in a way to keep each component in its reduced form. Lester Packer, head of the Packer Lab at the University of California has published over 700 papers and seventy books about antioxidants and health. This includes studies on the multiple actions of ALA in the body. In addition to the redox cycling of vitamins C and E, ALA raises the levels of the essential intracellular antioxidant glutathione and modulates signal transduction by NF-kappa B referred to above.[8,9] The human antioxidant system has multiple interactive and essential components. This may explain the negative outcome found occasionally in clinical studies using single antioxidants such as vitamin E.

Excitotoxicity is closely related to oxidative injury in neurologic disease. Russell Blaylock M.D., a neurosurgeon in Mississippi, deserves credit for bringing excitotoxicity to the public's attention, particularly related to external excitotoxins such as aspartame and monosodium glutamate (MSG).[10] Excitotoxicity literally means the toxic effect of exciting nerves' cells beyond their normal physiologic capacity. Dr. Blaylock based his work on numerous studies documenting the neurotoxic effects of MSG, and to a lesser degree, aspartame. [11,12,13] Aspartame consists of two amino acids, L-aspartic acid and L-phenylalanine, enfolded in a molecule L-aspartyl-L-phenylalanine-methyl ester. Although the literature on aspartame is less clear-cut, its relation to the excitatory metabolites L-aspartic acid and L-phenylalanine as well as the breakdown product methanol, suggests its danger for human consumption. Avoidance of MSG and aspartame is strongly recommended, particularly in individuals with neurologic illness.

Excitotoxicity also includes the effects of our own neurotransmitters, glutamate and, to a much lesser degree, dopamine.[14] There is evidence to implicate an excitotoxic role of glutamate in all the disorders discussed in this book. As will be discussed, some protection against glutamate toxicity may be provided by the use of branched chain amino acids and taurine. From a broader perspective, the protection of brain cells, or neuroprotection, against excitotoxicity as well as other insults is an important goal, particularly for individuals already affected by neurologic disorders. This is not simply alternative medicine, but has become a goal of mainstream neuroscience research.[15] Fortunately, a number of herbs and nutrients have documented neuroprotective value. These are addressed individually in this book as they relate to particular neurologic disorders.

It has become common knowledge that our planet is increasingly toxic. Perhaps the first individual to get the public's attention was Rachel Louise Carson, a writer, scientist and ecologist who died in 1964. She was Editor-in-Chief of all publications for the U.S. Fish and Wildlife Service. Disturbed by the indiscriminate use of synthetic pesticides, in 1962 she published *Silent Spring*, describing in detail how DDT entered the food chain, ultimately causing cancer and genetic damage. There are now literally hundreds of books related to environmental toxicity and health issues. More than 77,000 chemicals are being manufactured in North America with 3,000 added directly to our food supply. Over 10,000 chemicals are used in solvents, emulsifiers and preservatives in the food industry. The average city water supply contains over 500 chemicals. Many chemicals are not metabolized in the body and are stored in body fat. Most individuals demonstrate 400 to 800 different chemical residues in their fat cells. It is estimated that as high as 95% of cancers are related to diet and environmental toxicity. The Environmental Protection Agency has conducted the National Human Adipose Tissue Survey since 1976. Five toxic chemicals – OCDD (a dioxin derived from incineration of municipal and private waste), styrene (from the production and use of polystyrene plastics), 1,4-dichlorobenzene (household insecticide), xylene (automobile exhaust and painting materials), and ethylphenol – were found in 100% of samples. Another nine chemicals – benzene (industrial processes and automobile exhaust), toluene (gasoline, solvents, and tobacco), chlorobenzene (industrial and municipal discharges), ethylbenzene (numerous household products and manufacturing processes), DDE (pesticides), three dioxins and one furan (from thermal degradation of organic compounds) – were found in 91-98% of samples and a total of twenty toxic compounds were found in 76% of all samples. These chemicals affect the immune and endocrine system as well as the nervous system.

Toxic exposure has been implicated in four of the diseases discussed in this book. PD is the best studied with epidemiologic,[16,17] experimental,[18] and theoretical[19] evidence. A study at the Environmental and Occupational Health Sciences Institute of the University of Medicine and Dentistry of New Jersey demonstrated the toxic effects of the combination of the pesticides paraquat and maneb on the substantia nigra in the brainstem. Postnatal exposure of mice to paraquat and maneb resulted in permanent and selective loss of dopaminergic nerve cells in the substantia nigra pars compacta, the area affected in PD. Of further interest is that exposure to maneb alone during gestation markedly increased the toxicity to paraquat in adult mice.[20] This demonstrates the threshold effect of toxic environmental compounds. Initially the brain can compensate for the toxic effect with reserve capacity until ultimately a threshold is reached beyond which the compensation cannot occur and disease ensues. This hypothesis is rather vividly supported by multiple studies demonstrating increased levels of organochlorine pesticides in brains of PD patients.[21,22]

Exciting breakthroughs have occurred in understanding the role of neurotoxicity in PD. Discussed further in the PD chapter, the protein alpha-synuclein, which plays an essential role in neurophysiology, accumulates excessively in PD and is the main component of the abnormal inclusions, Lewy bodies. Proteins are catabolized and eliminated through two systems in every cell, the lysosomal system and the proteasome. The cylindrically shaped proteasome contains protein-degrading enzymes. A recent study confirmed that the proteasome is inhibited by maneb.[23] Since alpha-synuclein is metabolized by the proteasome, impairment of proteasomal function would result in alpha-synuclein accumulation. In addition, aggregated alpha-synuclein itself binds to and inhibits the proteasome, resulting in a positive feedback acceleration of toxicity.[24] Pesticides, such as rotenone, inhibit mitochondrial complex I, the first essential step in oxidative phosphorylation which creates the energy molecules adenosine triphosphate (ATP) from food. PD is known to have reduced complex I function. A recent German study found that complex I inhibition by rotenone resulted in lowered testosterone levels, postulated to contribute to PD.[25]

Environmental neurotoxins may play a role in the other disorders discussed in this book. A significant amount of work, particularly in Israel, has elucidated the importance of paraoxonase in atherosclerotic disease. Paraoxonase is an esterase enzyme located in tissue and on the surface of high-density lipoprotein (HDL) particles. It hydrolyzes organophosphate insecticides as well as arachidonic acid derivatives found on the surface of oxidized low-density lipoprotein (LDL) particles. Oxidized LDL particles may initiate the atherosclerotic lesions. There are three genes on chromosome 7 responsible for paraoxonase 1,2 and 3 (PON 1,2 and 3). PON1 and 3 are inactivated under oxidative stress (which occurs with neurotoxicity).[26] There are genetic variations in the PON gene cluster, presumably resulting in PON more or less effective in hydrolyzing toxins and the inflammatory compounds on the surface of LDL particles. Since paraoxonase is located on the surface of HDL particles, this genetic polymorphism would determine the ability of HDL particles to protect LDL particles from oxidative damage.[27] This would help explain hereditary influences on the development of atherosclerosis in relationship to toxic exposure.

Although less robust, a relationship exists between pesticide exposure and AD and MS. A French study found a 2.3 increase in risk for AD in elderly individuals with occupational exposure to pesticides.[28] Another French study showed a definite cognitive loss in individuals with occupational, low-level exposure to pesticides.[29] The threshold effect mentioned above suggests that these individuals may well have a greater risk for developing AD. An association also exists between solvent exposure and MS. Toxins may enhance pro-inflammatory responses including TNF-α and IL-1 cytokine production, molecules detrimental in MS.[30]

Heavy metal exposure is an increasingly dangerous health issue. The struggle to contain heavy metal toxicity extends from politics to biology. On the political side, relaxation of conditions that trigger the New Source Review provision of the Clean Air Act may increase environmental heavy metal burden. Although the significance of this has been questioned by the National Center for Policy Analysis (NCPA), a nonprofit, public policy research organization, there is no controversy regarding the cumulative burden of heavy metal burden and toxicity. Mercury, for example, will circulate in the atmosphere for years after industrial emission. Despite natural processes that might bury, dilute, or erode mercury deposits in localized areas, mercury concentrations in feathers of fish-eating seabirds from the northeastern Atlantic have steadily increased for over a century. Continued atmospheric deposition has gradually increased concentrations in otherwise pristine areas.[31] The mercury content of fish has reached such a level that the U.S. Environmental Protection Agency (EPA) has issued advisories for women who may become pregnant, are pregnant or are nursing. The EPA advises against eating shark, swordfish, king mackerel, and tilefish and restricting weekly intake of other fish, such as salmon, to 12oz/week. For fish caught locally without any mercury advisories, only 6oz/week are recommended.

The literature relating heavy metal exposure to four of the disorders discussed here is variably inconclusive and somewhat contradictory. Some relationships, though, are more definitive. A recent Finnish study demonstrated a 1.6 times greater incidence of coronary ischemic events in men with high hair mercury levels.[32] An article from Harvard Medical school in 2003 notes that the high mercury content in cold-water fish negates the diminished risk of coronary artery disease from fish consumption. They found that the mercury levels in five over-the-counter fish oils was negligible and suggested that supplementation with fish oil may provide a safer alternative to fish consumption.[33] In regards to PD, epidemiologic studies show a definitely increased risk with metal exposure[34,35] and an experimental study at University of California, Santa Cruz demonstrated that low levels of aluminum, copper, iron, cobalt, and manganese directly induced alpha-synuclein fibril formation.[36] Deposition of alpha-synuclein is considered part of the pathologic process in PD. Heavy metal exposure may play a role in MS. A study in 1994 revealed that lead increased the immunogenicity of myelin basic protein and glial fibrillary acidic protein with the production of autoantibodies against these proteins.[37] The experimental animal model for MS is created via the immune reaction to the injection of myelin basic protein. A paper in 2004 revealed a 1.24 times risk of developing MS in individuals with a significant amount of dental amalgam.[38] Dental amalgam is 50% elemental mercury in composition and its continued use is a subject of heated controversy. Dentists now appear to be switching to the use of composite (resin). A very recent German article on amalgam concluded with: "Summing up, available data suggests that dental amalgam is an unsuitable material for medical, occupational and ecological reasons.[39] Finally, AD may be related in part to mercury exposure. Some studies reveal elevated mercury levels in brains of deceased patients with AD and elevated blood levels in living patients. Apolipoprotein E4, a risk factor for AD may have reduced binding of mercury allowing a higher free fraction to enter the brain. A German article in 2004 concluded with: "In sum, both the findings from epidemiological and demographical studies, the frequency of amalgam application in industrialized countries, clinical studies, experimental studies, and the dental state of AD patients in comparison to controls suggest a decisive role for inorganic mercury in the etiology of AD.[40]

Mitochondrial dysfunction is an essential element in all the disorders. The nature of the dysfunction differs from one disorder to another. In particular, irreversible dysfunction in the degenerative disorders may actually lead to apoptosis, or cell death. Dysfunction in migraine appears to lead to a reduced threshold for the onset of headache. Although more benign in nature, the mitochondrial dysfunction in migraine can contribute to the episodically disabling nature of this condition.

We offer *Integrated Medicine for Neurologic Disorders* as an introduction to the vast naturopathic literature regarding these common neurologic disorders. Much of this literature appears in mainstream, peer-reviewed specialty journals, yet the implications remain unintegrated into standard medical practice. This is a loss for the patient, the practitioner, and the practice of medicine as a whole. The patient loses the benefit of simple, inexpensive remedies, and medicine itself becomes increasingly technical, expensive, and unavailable to all. A truly integrated medicine cannot afford to ignore any potential treatment because of financial, political, or paradigmatic reasons. We all lose in the end, encumbered by an increasingly expensive and less effective system of medicine.

The wisest mind has something yet to learn.
—George Santayana

Chapter One

Multiple Sclerosis

Multiple sclerosis (MS) is an autoimmune disease that affects the central nervous system (CNS). In America there currently are over 400,000 diagnosed cases. Myelin, a fatty tissue that surrounds nerve fibers and is essential for their function, is lost in different regions of the brain, spinal cord, or optic nerves as a result of the disease. This causes dysfunction in the signals being transmitted throughout the nervous system and can result in a wide range of unpredictable symptoms such as fatigue, depression, difficulty walking, dizziness, numbness, memory problems, bowel/bladder disturbances, sexual function changes, vision problems, or pain. Symptoms vary significantly between individuals and can change over time. MS generally occurs as episodic relapses or a slowly progressive course. Although the ultimate cause is unknown, it has definite autoimmune features including a reduction in suppressor lymphocytes during attacks and an increase in the proinflammatory cytokines, interferon (IFN)-gamma and tumor necrosis factor-alpha (TNF-α).

Two new agents, IFN-beta-Ib (Betaseron, 0.25mg subcutaneously every other day) and IFN-beta-Ia (Avonex, 30mcg intramuscular once/week), appear to inhibit release of

IFN-gamma and tumor necrosis factor (TNF), partially restore suppressor cell function, and attenuate disease activity. There is approximately a 30% reduction in relapse rate with these agents and a reduction in new lesions, as shown on patient magnetic resonance imaging (MRI) films. Unfortunately, after twenty-four months of treatment, 40% and 16% of patients treated with IFN-beta Ib and IFN-beta Ia respectively, develop neutralizing antibodies. Neutralizing antibodies are proteins produced by the body to block the effect of the drug. A newer agent, Copaxone (glatiramer acetate), is the acetate salt of synthetic polypeptides containing four naturally occurring amino acids, L-glutamic acid, L-alanine, L-tyrosine and L-lysine. It reduces the incidence of experimental allergic encephalomyelitis (EAE), the animal model of MS. It appears to reduce the immune reaction to myelin, stimulate lymphocytes to release anti-inflammatory signaling molecules, and stimulate the release of a trophic, or nurturing, substance for brain cells called brain-derived neurotrophic factor (BDNF). Patients treated with Copaxone have approximately 30% fewer relapses.[41] Additionally, there are significantly fewer side effects as compared with the interferons mentioned above. Antibodies do develop that react with Copaxone but do not appear to diminish its efficacy. Copaxone dosage is 20mg/day subcutaneously.

Health issues in MS are part of a larger set of problems facing the population as a whole.[42] All of the problems mentioned below have been shown to be particularly salient in the development or progression of MS.

- **Pervasive deficiency of essential nutrients related to non-sustainable agriculture and the loss of nutrients in our food:** According to *The Healing Power of Minerals* (Paul Bergner, Prima Publishing,

1997), charts from the U.S. Department of Agriculture document a greater than 80% drop in the mineral content of vegetables from 1914 compared with 1997. We have lost a significant percentage of our topsoil as well as the humus layer, the portion of the soil that contains the minerals and other nutrients essential to human health. Often, fruits and vegetables are picked before they ripen, and before flavonoids and other important nutrients have a chance to reach the concentrations present in vine ripened fruit and vegetables. Readers interested in studying these issues in more depth are referred to Mr. Berger's excellent book. Up to 50% of the population fails to ingest the recommended daily allowance (RDA) for essential vitamins and minerals. One solution is to buy organic foods, which contain higher levels of vitamins and minerals and are farmed using sustainable methods that support the environment.

- **Diets deficient in essential fatty acids due to the use of processed foods, margarine, and refined grains:** Many processed foods transform the normal cis form of fatty acids to the toxic trans form. These are called trans fats and hydrogenated or partially-hydrogenated oils, and have been proven to cause disease even in very small amounts.[43] It is essential to check food labels and avoid all products containing trans fats or hydrogenated oils.

- **Exposure to increasing levels of oxidation:** This is related to loss of atmospheric protection (ozone hole), increased oxidative toxins in the environment (pesticides, pollution), and diminished endogenous antioxidants (those that reside in the body).

- **Increasing exposure to a toxic environment:** Heavy metals such as lead from pesticide sprays and cooking utensils; cadmium and lead from cigarette smoke; mercury from dental fillings, contaminated fish, and cosmetics; and aluminum from antacids, antiperspirants, and cookware pose significant health hazards and must be avoided.

- **Diminished gastrointestinal health:** The use of antibiotics, non-steroidal anti-inflammatories such as ibuprofen or naproxen, and other drugs cause changes in intestinal microflora and the viability of the intestinal wall. This can lead to intestinal dysbiosis, an imbalance in the gut bacteria, and intestinal permeability syndrome, the passage of toxic substances across the gut wall due to damage to the protective barrier. Reduction in use of these medications when possible and according to physician recommendation, and increased intake of foods with active cultures (L. acidopilus, B. bifidus, S. thermophilus, L. bulgaricus, and L. casie), such as yogurt, can improve gastrointestinal health. Probiotics, supplements containing beneficial bacteria, may also be helpful.

- **Increased excitotoxicity and inflammation:** Consuming products containing ingredients such as monosodium glutamate (MSG), hydrolyzed vegetable protein, or aspartame can lead to over stimulation and lethal injury of nerve cells. This process, excitotoxicity, contributes to the progression of MS. Inflammation also plays a role in MS and can be addressed with herbs and nutrients discussed below.

Specific Dietary and Nutritional Supplements in Multiple Sclerosis

Diet: Epidemiology confirms that MS is directly correlated to diets high in animal and dairy products, which contain saturated fats. This was first proposed by Dr. Ray Swank in 1950[44] and supported by a number of subsequent studies including a Norwegian study in 1952[45] as well as later studies.[46,47] These early observations were the first to attempt to explain the strong increase in MS with latitude, suggesting the correlation was due to the fact that people in colder climates often consume more fat in their diet. The Norwegian study, in particular, emphasized the critical importance of certain essential fats in the development of MS. The people living inland, with diets high in land animal fat, had eight times the incidence of MS as the people living on the coast, with diets consisting of a large amount of fish.

In 1956, Sinclair suggested that a deficient intake of polyunsaturated fatty acids might explain the epidemiological findings linking MS incidence to diet.[48] Subsequently, reduced levels of a polyunsaturated fatty acid, linoleic acid, were found in MS patients in serum, erythrocytes, lymphocytes and platelets.[49] A meta-analysis of three linoleic acid studies revealed that patients with minor disability at study entry who were treated with linoleic acid supplementation showed less deterioration than controls. The study also showed a reduction in severity and duration of relapses associated with linoleic acid treatment.[50] A Norwegian study performed in 2000[51] involved sixteen patients and a daily supplement of 5ml of fish oil containing 400mg of eicosapentaenoic acid (EPA) and 500mg of docosahexaenoic acid (DHA), two important essential polyunsaturated fatty acids. The patients also received 3333

IU of vitamin A, 400IU of vitamin D, and approximately 5.5 IU/day of vitamin E. The patients were advised to reduce intake of sugar, coffee, tea, alcohol, and saturated fat from meat and dairy products. They also were advised to increase their consumption of fish, fruit, vegetables, and whole grain bread. It should be noted that alcohol increases the proinflammatory prostaglandin 2 series in the body, which could exacerbate the inflammatory process in MS. Compared with their baseline status, the annual exacerbation rate fell 96% and disability scores fell 25% on the Expanded Disability Status Scale (EDSS). Of the sixteen patients, eleven improved, four remained the same, and only one deteriorated during the two-year period. The two patients who had a relapse during the study continued to smoke. This is a striking, albeit uncontrolled study. It confirms Dr. Swank's uncontrolled study over thirty-four years of 144 patients on a low saturated fat diet, supplemented with polyunsaturated fat, who did significantly better than that expected from the general MS population.[52] Although criticized for a lack of a control group, Swank himself notes that in a study of this length, a control group would have been highly impractical, if not unethical. His outcome figures, though, can be compared to general epidemiological figures for MS prognosis, which would suggest that a diet low in saturated fats and high in polyunsaturated fats is beneficial for MS patients. His recommended daily diet included 5gm of cod liver oil and 10-40gm of vegetable oil, and limited saturated fat to less than 20gm. He notes though that patients consuming 10-15gm/day of saturated fat had even better improvement in energy.

Essential fatty acids, a dietary requirement not produced in the body, have multiple effects that may explain their benefit for MS. EPA and DHA reduce a number of proinflammatory substances in the body including prostaglandin E2, substances secreted by white blood cells including leukotriene B4, and other proinflammatory cytokines. In addition, EPA and DHA are precursors to the anti-inflammatory prostaglandin 3 series. DHA may be the most critical essential fatty acid for nerve cell membranes, including myelin, the coating around nerves, which degenerates in MS. It is particularly critical during infant and childhood development because deficiency is associated with developmental cognitive and visual impairment. The critical importance of essential fatty acids, particularly DHA, during development may help explain why people from high risk areas, moving to low risk areas before the age of fifteen, take on an MS risk of the low risk area and vice versa.

In summary, saturated fat intakes should be limited to 10-20gm/day. This can be accomplished through reduction of animal fats other than those found in fish. Fish, high in omega-3 fatty acids, should be eaten at least three times/week. Due to the deficiency in omega-6 and omega-3 fatty acids in the general public and in MS patients in particular, the diet should be supplemented with essential fatty acids. Research suggests MS patients may experience a reduction in frequency and severity of relapses with omega-3 and omega-6 fatty acid supplementation.[53] Studies show that the omega-3 and omega-6 fatty acids compete for the same metabolic enzymes, and that our food supply has shifted from those rich in omega-3 to omega-6 because of the increased shelf life of omega-6 oils. Rather than a healthy 4:1 ratio of omega-6:omega-3 fatty acid intake, most Americans currently consume a diet with a 20:1 ratio. The omega-6 fatty acids give rise to both the anti-inflammatory prostaglandin 1 series and the proinflammatory prostaglandin 2 series. The omega-3 fatty acids give rise to the anti-inflammatory prostaglandin 3 series. We need all the prostaglandins but it is important to balance our intake to favor the anti-inflammatory series. A

4:1 ratio of omega-6:omega-3 intake is recommended. Flaxseed oil is high in omega-3 fatty acids. Unfortunately, we only convert about 3% of the linolenic acid in flaxseed oil to DHA, an important essential fatty acid. DHA and EPA are found in fish oil, and reduce the formation of the proinflammatory prostaglandin 2 series.[54] Dosage is approximately 500-1000mg/day of DHA plus EPA and can be taken in gel-capsule form. It is important to take oil from fish that lived in unpolluted waters; those free from heavy metals and pesticide residues. The label on the bottle should make reference to assays showing no heavy metals or pesticide residues. Carlson's Norwegian Cod Liver Oil and Nordic Naturals provide such products. Some supplementation with omega-6 fatty acid, and gamma linoleic acid (GLA) in particular, may be warranted in individuals eating a highly non-processed, organic diet. GLA is an omega-6 fatty acid found in borage oil, black currant seed, oil and evening primrose oil. Dosage for omega-6 fatty acids is a combined total 250mg/day of GLA plus linoleic acid.

Glutathione: Due to reduced activity of glutathione peroxidase (GP), an important enzyme in the body's antioxidant system, MS patients have a reduced capacity to detoxify free radicals.[55] In the body, GP transforms dangerous peroxides, such as hydrogen and lipid peroxides, into harmless molecules. Lipid peroxide, formed through the oxidation of myelin lipids, is dangerous because it destroys myelin. In a recent study, measurements of GP in the spinal fluid of MS patients showed patients had reduced GP levels compared to controls.[56] These, as well as other studies, suggest a role of oxidative stress in the cause or aggravation of MS.[57,58]

GP has a selenium dependent and a selenium independent form. Selenium is an essential trace mineral that is important for the function of the immune system and antioxidant enzymes. A 1988 study appears to confirm a selenium deficiency in MS patients, correlating with the known oxidative disorder in MS.[59] This report, as well as a more recent study,[60] shows that these deficits in the MS patient can be safely reversed with antioxidant supplementation. The latter study supplemented patients with selenium and vitamins C and E. The prior study used only selenium. Vitamin E, a fat-soluble antioxidant, is very important in protecting myelin, particularly if the individual is increasing their polyunsaturated fat intake. The extra essential fatty acids will require additional antioxidant protection in the body. These studies stress the importance of antioxidant supplementation in MS. Vitamin E dosage is 200-600 IU/day, selenium up to 200mcg/day, and vitamin C up to 1000mg/day. It is important to use d-alpha tocopherol, the natural form of vitamin E. Also, it is essential to use a product that contains mixed tocopherols, the class of molecules constituting vitamin E, which may be as important if not more important than alpha-tocopherol for certain functions in the body.

GP requires glutathione (GSH), a triplet of the amino acids glutamate, cysteine and glycine, to function. GSH is poorly absorbed orally, but can be supported indirectly by antioxidants such as alpha-lipoic acid (ALA), a powerful fat- and water-soluble antioxidant that works both inside and outside of cells and easily crosses the blood-brain barrier. It is synthesized in the liver and other tissues. Because it is fat soluble, it can protect against the lipid peroxidation of myelin. Studies also reveal an improvement in mitochondrial function with ALA. The mitochondria generate the energy in cells, including nerve cells. Healthy energy production is necessary for many nerve cell functions including protection against toxic damage. ALA helps regenerate the reduced active forms of vitamins C and E and increases GSH levels. It also helps protect against mercury and lead toxicity, an increasing problem today. ALA is rapidly cleared from the blood with a half-life of about thirty minutes. For this reason, a sustained release form of 300mg/day is recommended.

The sulfur containing amino acid, N-acetyl cysteine (NAC), is antioxidant, helps detoxify the body of heavy metals and toxic environmental compounds, increases GSH levels, and decreases tumor necrosis-alpha (TNF-α), levels. TNF, a cytokine, or information molecule, secreted by white blood cells, is significantly elevated in MS, which in turn results in increased free radical formation. In addition, TNF induces special molecules on the cells lining the cerebral blood vessels, called adhesion molecules, which aid the migration of inflammatory white blood cells into the brain.[61] A study in Israel demonstrated that NAC significantly reduced the occurrence of acute EAE.[62] Finally, NAC appears to reduce various members of a class of enzymes called matrix metaloproteinases (MMPs), found pervasively in the body.[63,64] Their normal function is the scavenging of dead matter essential to wound healing and tissue growth. There is evidence of increased MMPs in patients with MS. This may facilitate the passage of inflammatory cells into the CNS as well as increase the degradation of myelin and axons (nerve fibers).[65,66] We are not aware of any clinical studies to date, measuring the effects of NAC in MS. Based on the information presented above and the safety of NAC, NAC is recommended in MS at a dosage of 500mg twice/day on an empty stomach.

Patients should also be aware of the potential benefits of phosphatidylserine (PS), the major acidic fatty substance (phospholipid) in brain cell membranes. In addition to reducing cortisol in chronically stressed individuals and increasing brain neurotransmitters, PS inhibits the release of

TNF. A study at Albert Einstein College of Medicine revealed that PS significantly reduced the occurrence of EAE in mice.[67] The recommended PS dosage is 300mg/day.

Vitamin B12: British neurologists have reported a vitamin B12 deficiency in a significant percentage of MS patients.[68] Another study showed that lower vitamin B12 levels were seen in patients whose MS started prior to age eighteen.[69] Vitamin B12 deficiency is associated with demyelination of the CNS. The vitamin is involved in methylation processes, adding a methyl group (a carbon and 4 hydrogens) to proteins and other substances. It appears essential in the methylation of myelin basic protein, an important protein in myelin. Vitamin B12 then is essential to the formation and repair of myelin, the tissue damaged by inflammation in MS.

Of interest is a study by Goodkin and others in which they found low vitamin B12 values in thirty-two of 156 MS patients but found elevated levels of homocysteine and methylmalonic acid (MMA) in only seven of these patients.[70] These compounds accumulate in vitamin B12 deficiency since their metabolizing enzymes require vitamin B12 as a co-factor. Goodkin and his co-authors concluded that the vitamin B12 deficiency in MS may not be clinically significant. On the other hand, MS patients may have a subtler problem, such as a CNS transport disorder of vitamin B12, occurring in the setting when the role of vitamin B12 in the metabolism of homocysteine and MMA is normal. One study showed reduced ratios of serum:cerebrospinal fluid vitamin B12 levels in MS, supporting the concept of a problem transporting vitamin B12 into the CNS in MS.[71] A Japanese study in 1994 involved giving 60mg/day of methylcobalamin to six patients with chronic progressive MS for six months. There was an improvement in the visual and brainstem evoked responses although no improvement in motor disability.[72] Although baseline vitamin B12 levels were normal in the study, there was a significant decrease in the unsaturated vitamin B12 binding capacities.

There is no toxicity to vitamin B12 and evidence supports supplementation in MS. The usual vitamin B12 oral supplement is cyanocobalamin, which the body converts in the liver to methylcobalamin. Because of the recommended high dosage of 1-2mg/day, methylcobalamin is the preferred form of the supplement. This is available from Thorne, a supplement manufacturer.

It should be noted that three other B vitamins – B6, niacin, and riboflavin – are important in myelin formation. Supplementation is recommended in the form of a high quality vitamin-mineral supplement containing approximately 10mg of vitamin B6, 150mg of niacin, and 10mg of riboflavin.

Vitamin D: One of the more important scientific discoveries recently involves the role of vitamin D deficiency in MS. An initial study in 1994 found inadequate vitamin D levels in eighty female MS patients in New York. This was correlated with reduced bone mineral density in these patients.[73] A subsequent study showed that the hormonally active form of vitamin D prevented EAE.[74] This suggested that vitamin D was a hormonal regulator of the immune system. In addition, decreasing sunlight from the equator would result in diminished vitamin D levels, which is dependent on sunlight. This gradient in sunlight would correlate with the increasing incidence of MS with distance from the equator. Vitamin D levels would also explain the disparity of MS incidence in Switzerland with high rates at low altitudes and low rates at high altitudes, because ultraviolet light intensity, responsible for vitamin D formation rates, is higher at higher altitudes. Vitamin D concentration would also explain the low incidence on the Norwegian coast and the higher incidence inland. Fish oils are high in vitamin D and fish is a staple for the Norwegian coastal people. The inland Norwegians rely on land animal meat as a staple in their diet. The authors concluded: " … MS may be preventable in genetically susceptible individuals with early intervention strategies that provide adequate levels of hormonally active 1,25-dihydroxyvitamin D3 or its analog."[75]

The active form of vitamin D is now known to have immunoregulatory properties. It inhibits the production of interleukin-12 (IL12), a substance secreted by lymphocytes and known to be involved in the development of autoimmune diseases, such as MS. Vitamin D also stimulates the production of two anti-inflammatory substances (cytokines) secreted by white blood cells, interleukin-4 and transforming growth factor beta-1. A study done in 2000 showed that a vitamin D3 analogue prevented the chronic relapsing form of EAE.[76] A second study confirmed that vitamin D3 partially prevented EAE and decreased macrophage accumulation in the CNS of the experimental animals.[77] Macrophages are the white blood cells that consume the myelin fragments in an MS attack.

Based on the above information, vitamin D supplementation is recommended in MS. To ensure adequate serum levels, a total supply of 100mcg (4000IU) is recommended. In fact, there are no adverse effects from a daily supply of 250mcg (10,000IU) the amount received from total-body sun exposure in one day. Known cases of toxicity with hypercalcemia all involved intakes equal or greater than 1000mcg/day.[78]

Pineal gland and melatonin: A tiny structure at the base of the brain, the pineal gland, secretes a sleep-regulating hormone called melatonin. The pineal gland may play a role in MS. A recent study showed a positive correlation between nocturnal melatonin levels and older age of onset as well as a negative correlation between melatonin levels and duration of illness.[79] In other words, higher melatonin levels may provide a protective effect against MS. Of interest is that during pregnancy, melatonin levels are high and drop just before delivery. This correlates with the drop in incidence of MS relapses during pregnancy and the rise after delivery.[80] It is also of interest that melatonin secretion varies with the season, menstrual cycle, and the onset of puberty and menopause. It modulates the circadian rhythms of the immune system and appears to influence myelination in the CNS. These observations may explain a number of epidemiologic facts about MS including its variation with latitude and the change in incidence relative to developmental stages such as puberty and menopause. Based on these studies, a small amount of melatonin, between 0.2-1mg at bedtime, appears warranted.

Antigen-antibody complexes: In MS there is evidence for increased circulating antigen-antibody complexes, mediators of immune responses. Reductions in circulating complexes correlate with clinical improvement. Supplements that reduce them include plant derived proteolytic enzymes, bromelain, and papain. A number of supplements use various combinations of different enzymes. Suggested dosage for pancreatin is 350-700mg three times/day between meals using a 10X preparation. Bromelain, an extract from pineapple, interrupts the body's inflammatory pathway in several ways. The authors are not aware of a controlled study of bromelain in MS; however, its anti-inflammatory properties and its safety suggest its consideration for MS patients. A typical bromelain dosage is 2400GDU two-four times/day on an empty stomach. Follow the directions on the bottle for the papain dosage. For a combination product, use the dosage recommended by the manufacturer.

Maldigestion and malabsorption: Studies indicate that a significant percentage of MS patients have some degree of maldigestion and malabsorption.[81] Diminished fat absorption, poor meat digestion, and poor vitamin B12 absorption was found to be 42%, 41%, and 12%, respectively, in a group of MS patients. This study also found vitamin A and carotene levels to be at the lowest limit of normal in the majority of patients. A microscopic study of jejunal (small intestine) biopsies revealed measles virus antigens, complement (an important cascade of proteins activated in inflammation), and probable antigen-antibody complex deposition. An earlier study revealed fine structural abnormalities in six to eight jejunal biopsies in MS patients, which would correlate with problems with malabsorption.[82] Malabsorption will lead to nutrient deficiencies that may aggravate the disease process. In addition, maldigestion, or putrefaction of food, leads to toxic products in the bowel that injure the bowel wall and increase its permeability to pathogenic microorganisms and toxic chemicals. This stresses the immune system, increases oxidative stress, and could well aggravate the disease. If the individual has any symptoms of improper digestion, then plant digestive enzymes and nutrient products designed to heal the gut wall should be considered. Tyler makes an excellent line of these products.

Infections: Infection has long been considered as a cause or at least an associated phenomenon of MS. As noted by Dr. Perlmutter, by 1998, at least sixteen agents have been considered.[83] The most recent agent is Chlamydia pneumoniae, a bacterium that causes upper respiratory illness and may be related to a type of arthritis and coronary artery disease. In 1999, researchers at Vanderbilt School of Medicine found immunological evidence for this bacterium in the spinal fluid of 97% of MS patients versus only 18% of controls.[84] A subsequent study in Heidelberg, Germany found a much lower incidence of evidence in the cerebrospinal fluid of MS patients.[85] A recent study did not find evidence for this bacteria in the brain lesions of deceased MS patients.[86] Unfortunately, this pattern of events in MS studies has occurred commonly in the search for an infectious agent of MS. Other recent potentially associated organisms include Candida albicans and Human Herpes Virus 6. Due to the lack of confirmatory evidence, treatment of an individual with MS for an infectious organism should be on a case-by-case basis. If evidence for Chlamydia pneumoniae is found, for example, then treatment with an antibiotic such as doxycycline should be considered.

Glycine: By inhibiting the motor reflex arc in the spinal cord, glycine controls spasticity. Threonine is a potential precursor of glycine that crosses the blood-brain barrier. A study at Massachusetts General Hospital showed that 7.5gm/day of threonine reduced signs of spasticity on examination, although there was no symptomatic improvement. There were no side effects of the threonine, recommending its potential use in MS patients.[87] Threonine dosage per this study is 7.5gm/day.

Magnesium: An autopsy study in Japan revealed a significant reduction in magnesium levels in the CNS as well as other organs in MS patients. The most marked reduction was in the white matter of the brain, the location of MS plaques.[88] Magnesium is essential to the function of the N-methyl-D-aspartate (NMDA) receptor, the nerve cell receptor for the excitatory neurotransmitter glutamate. A deficiency of magnesium enhances the effect of glutamate, resulting in a calcium influx into the nerve cell, damaging the cell. Magnesium is also essential for the proper functioning of adenosine triphosphate (ATP), the main energy molecule of the body, and is involved in hundreds of different chemical reactions in the body. Magnesium supplementation is at least 200mg twice/day. Magnesium can cause diarrhea when taken without calcium. To avoid this, and particularly in older women who need calcium supplementation, at least 400mg of calcium is recommended along with the magnesium.

Inosine: Inosine is a purine, a type of molecule found in DNA. It is found in plants, animals and other living matter. It is closely related to another purine, adenosine, and a 2002 study revealed that it increased intracellular ATP levels.[89] ATP is the energy storage molecule in the body. Inosine is also an intermediate in the degradation of purines to their end products, uric acid.

Multiple studies have shown reduced uric acid levels in MS patients and little if any overlap of gout and MS.[90,91] This is significant because gout occurs in conditions of high uric acid levels. In addition, patients having relapses of MS have lower uric acid levels than those in remission, and those with a disrupted blood-brain barrier had lower levels as well. Uric acid is a scavenger of peroxynitrite, one of the most dangerous free radicals in the body. Peroxynitrite is derived from nitric oxide and the super-oxide radical and has been implicated in the pathogenesis of MS as well as EAE.[92] Also of note is that uric acid suppresses EAE in animals. This may relate to its anti-inflammatory effect, documented in a 2001 study. In this study, inosine suppressed the inflammatory effect of TNF and inhibited the creation of another proinflammatory substance, interleukin-8.[93] Another interesting fact about inosine is its ability to significantly enhance growth of nerve fibers (axons) in the CNS. There are multiple postulated mechanisms for this effect.[94]

The studies mentioned above suggest a benefit of using inosine to raise uric acid levels in MS patients. This may result in increased ATP levels, provide more energy for the patient, reduce peroxynitrite levels and reduce the free radical contribution to the progression of the disease. This can be accomplished by taking inosine, up to 5gm/day. Anecdotal reports suggest a dosage up to 500mg every two hours during active periods.[95] A study at the University of Pennsylvania concluded the mechanism of action of inosine treatment on EAE mice was through the metabolism of inosine to uric acid.[96] In another study, the same research group found three of eleven MS patients showed clinical improvement, and the remaining eight patients showed no disease progression, during a ten-month period after treatment with oral inosine.[97] They also found that oral administration of uric acid failed to raise serum uric acid levels, while oral administration of inosine raised uric acid levels with no side effects. Of interest is that Copaxone, a well-accepted immune modulator drug for MS, significantly raises uric acid levels. The interferon drugs do not appear to raise uric acid levels.[98] The only potential side effect is that elevated uric acid levels may cause gout. Uric acid levels should be measured prior to and during treatment. The supplement should be discontinued if gout symptoms appear. It should not be used in patients with kidney disease or gout.

Excitotoxicity and inflammation: There is increasing evidence for an abnormal process called excitotoxicity contributing to the progression of MS. Excitoxicity refers to the lethal injury of a nerve cell due to over stimulation. The excitation may be caused by our own neurotransmitters, such as glutamate, or by something we ingest, such as MSG, hydrolyzed vegetable protein, or aspartame. Elevated glutamate levels, a risk factor for excitotoxicity, have been correlated with MS pathology. MS patients have higher cerebrospinal fluid glutamate levels when they are having a relapse compared to when they are in their stable phase. Patients in their stable phase but with active lesions, detected radiologically, have higher cerebrospinal fluid glutamate levels than stable patients with no active lesions.[99] These elevated levels may occur because the ability to remove excess glutamate is impaired in MS patient white matter, part of the nervous system that is pathological in the disease.[100] An inability to maintain normal glutamate levels has been shown to contribute to this white matter pathology.[101,102] Several recent studies have shown that the mechanism for this damage to white matter in MS is excitotoxicity.[103,104,105,106]

MS also involves an autoimmune inflammatory reaction that results in nerve fiber (axon) damage and demyelination. The damage to axons and the myelin insulation of neurons is caused in part by inflammatory mediators, such as cytokines, prostaglandins, and TNF, which are produced by lymphocytes called T cells.[107,108,109,110] A recent study from the Neurovirology Research Laboratory in Salt Lake City provides important information connecting the roles of inflammation and excitotoxicity. The authors of this study concluded that glutamate-induced excitotoxic damage to oligodendrocytes, the myelin producing cells of the CNS, contribute to the lesions of MS.[111] The scientists also found that Cyclooxygenase-2 (COX-2) and nitric oxide synthase were expressed together in the lesions of MS. As discussed in the Parkinson's disease (PD) chapter, nitric oxide, created by the enzyme nitric oxide synthase, as well as COX-2, play key roles in inflammation and excitotoxic nerve cell injury. Further support that inflammation and excitotoxicity play intertwined roles in MS came from the results of a study suggesting that excitotoxicity, caused in part by high glutamate levels produced by activated immune cells, was one of the mechanisms underlying MS lesions during periods of inflammation.[112,113] Understanding that both inflammation and excitotoxicity play a role in MS can help a patient to maximize the beneficial use of herbs and nutrients.

Patients with MS need to reduce sources of excitotoxicity in the nervous system. It is important to eliminate MSG, hydrolyzed vegetable protein, and aspartame from the diet. These food additives are known excitotoxins. Supplementing with branched chain amino acids, L-leucine, L-isoleucine, and L-valine may help reduce excitotoxicity as they increase the metabolism of glutamate. Protein supplements, such as Spectrum Shake by Nutribiotic, contain branched chain amino acids. The amino acid taurine may also be helpful. It helps convert glutamate to the inhibitory neurotransmitter gamma-aminobutyric acid (GABA) and reduces the intracellular flux of calcium caused by glutamate. Taurine dosage is 500mg twice/day on an empty stomach.

A number of supplements reduce inflammation and specifically inhibit the COX-2 enzyme. A fuller explanation may be found in the section on inflammation in the PD chapter as well the introduction to the book. It is important to avoid simple sugars as they increase inflammation in multiple ways in the body. Of the many herbs that inhibit COX-2, turmeric extract, 900mg/day, may be the most effective. Of particular importance for MS, turmeric suppresses the effects of TNF, a known mediator of the MS disease mechanism.[114] The omega-3 fatty acids DHA and EPA, discussed in other parts of this chapter, are also anti-inflammatory. Dosage is 500-1000mg/day of the combination of EPA and DHA in liquid or gel capsules. Nordic Naturals and Carlson Laboratories are safe sources for fish oil, which needs to be free of detectable levels of pesticides and heavy metals. A small amount of GLA may be utilized. It generally comes with linoleic acid with a total dosage of both GLA and linoleic acid of 250mg/day. GLA is found in borage oil, black currant seed oil, and evening primrose oil. Another supplement that also may be helpful is bromelain, up to 2400 GDU (gelatin dissolving units) four times/day. Reduction of excitotoxicity and inflammation may be particularly important during an MS relapse.

Herbal supplements: MS activity and secondary symptoms, including spasticity, pain, insomnia, and bladder problems, may be reduced by treatment with herbal supplements, including those listed below.

● **Padma 28:** A number of countries, including Switzerland, Poland, Austria, Israel, and the United States have studied Padma 28, an herbal mixture of 25 herbal constituents combined in a specific order with strict weight ratios. Its efficacy in various disorders is related to modulation of immunological function. Several studies, including an Israeli study in 1995, suggest an anti-inflammatory effect.[115] Padma 28 inhibits lysozyme (a substance that breaks down tissue) release from stimulated human neutrophils and reduces nitric oxide production in macrophages. Nitric oxide is a small and pervasive molecule in the body that can be involved in inflammatory processes. Two of the constituents of Padma 28, costus root (the dried root of Saussurea chebula) and myrobalani fructus (the dried fruit of Terminalia chebula), by themselves inhibited nitric oxide production. A 1999 study in the U.S. showed that Padma 28 had a dose-dependent effect against EAE in mice.[116] Badmaev and his co-authors suggest that the protective effect could best be explained by a broad protective mechanism of action referred to as nonspecific resistance (NSR) to diverse biological and psychological stressors. The class of herbs or substances exhibiting these properties is called adaptogens or bioprotectants. A Polish study in 1982 showed improved suppressor cell function in T lymphocytes exposed to Padma 28.[117] Suppressor cells are a subset of lymphocytes involved in inhibiting inflammatory reactions. The study revealed improved differentiation and maturation of the suppressor cell subset of T lymphocytes.

Another study in Poland involved Padma treatment for twenty-nine relapsing and twenty-eight slowly progressive MS patients. Improvement occurred in 52% of the relapsing group with 10% showing deterioration and 38% remaining stable. In a similar control group, none improved, deterioration occurred in 35%, and 65% were stable. In the slowly progressive group, 33% enjoyed improvement, 14% worsened, and 52% were stable. In a similar control group, none improved, 47% deteriorated and the rest were stable. A third of the patients with abnormal visual evoked potentials (VEP) showed improvement in the VEP with Padma 28. There was no change in the auditory evoked potentials. The neurologic improvement in patients included a reduction in pyramidal, cerebellar and sphincter symptomatology. There were no side effects and routine blood tests did not reveal any changes in the study.[118] Padma 28 is available from Econugenics in the United States. Dosage is two tablets three times/day.

• **Ginkgo biloba:** Cerebral microcirculation and neurotransmitter levels are increased with the use of Ginkgo biloba, an antioxidant that also inhibits platelet aggregation. Relapses of MS are associated with inflammation, passage of white blood cells into the CNS, and damage to the blood-brain barrier. Platelet activating factor, inhibited by a compound in Ginkgo biloba called ginkgolide B, plays an important role in the vascular stage of inflammation. In addition, ginkgolide B can prevent and treat EAE. A multi-center, placebo-controlled study in France did not show a significant benefit from seven days of IV ginkgolide B but there was a trend in favor of the compound with a dose-effect relation.[119] A follow-up subgroup given gadolinium on serial MRI testing revealed some benefit of the ginkgolide B on reducing CNS lesions. Perhaps using other constituents of Ginkgo biloba, given according to a different protocol would result in more significant benefits. Given the multiple effects of Ginko biloba on the CNS and the results of this study, it should be considered for usage in MS at the standard dosage of 40mg three times/day or 60mg twice/day. Ginko biloba needs to be supplemented carefully when other platelet inhibitors or anticoagulants are being used. This includes the supplements vitamin E and essential fatty acids and the drugs coumadin, aspirin, Ticlid, and Aggrenox. In the presence of heart disease or stroke, or when an individual is on numerous medications, physician supervision should be available when using Ginkgo.

- **Other herbs:** St. John's Wort, which is anti-inflammatory, antimicrobial, and antidepressant should be considered for MS as it is also a vulnerary, or wound-healer, for the nervous system. Two Ayurvedic herbs, Ashwagandha and Bacopa, are antioxidant and have gentle restorative effects on the nervous system. Ashwagandha is the Indian equivalent to Ginseng, helping the individual adapt to stress. It also promotes sleep. Bacopa is noted to increase intellectual capacity. All these herbs may be beneficial in MS. Dosages are 300mg three times/day for St. John's Wort, 500mg twice/day for Ashwagandha, and 100mg twice/day with meals for Bacopa.

Additional modalities: A study has demonstrated that physical exercise benefits physical function, social interaction, emotional status and other measures in MS patients.[120] The value of exercise in MS has been problematic due to the prevalence of fatigue and concern regarding raising body temperature. On the other hand, aerobic exercise has shown substantial health benefits in various studies. This study involved fifteen weeks of aerobic training in MS patients and resulted in significant increases in muscle strength, a profound impact on quality of life with improved ambulation, mobility, and body-care as well as reduction in depression, anger, and fatigue. Based on this study, after appropriate medical clearance, MS patients should pursue a regular aerobic exercise program.

There are three studies showing benefit of acupuncture in MS including the treatment of associated trigeminal neuralgia and the reduction of spasticity.[121] Acupuncture, an ancient form of medical treatment based on Chinese medical theory, has a long scholarly tradition with numerous studies in many medical conditions. Studies satisfying statistical requirements of control, randomization, and blindedness are understandably difficult, if not impossible, to perform. As with all treatment modalities, including pharmaceutical ones, only a portion of patients respond. The safety and economy of acupuncture recommend it as a significant therapeutic option.

The benefits of imagery and cognitive therapy have been reported in two MS studies.[122,123] The use of imagery resulted in significant reductions in state anxiety and a stable internal locus of control while the control group shifted to a less internal locus of control. The multi-modal cognitive therapy study revealed significant improvements in verbal learning, verbal abstraction, depression, and, in some, measures of grip strength and tactile sensitivity. This study involved group psychotherapy, visualization techniques, guided imagery, meditation, relaxation, and mental and physical exercises.

Summary

Every MS patient is different, as is his or her disease. Only general recommendations can be made since each patient's needs will be different. Based on scientific evidence and our personal experience with MS patients, the following basic recommendations are suggested.

Diet: DHA and EPA can be obtained in gel-capsule form or as a liquid. Due to the FDA-confirmed problem with mercury toxicity in fish, an uncontaminated source of fish oil is recommended. Carlson Labs and Nordic Naturals both make safe and high quality fish oil products. In gel-capsule form, the combined dosage of DHA plus EPA should be up to 1gm/day. Some supplementation with GLA, an omega-6 fatty acid, may be beneficial, particularly in individuals eating a highly non-processed diet. Dosage is 250mg/day of GLA plus linoleic acid. Limit saturated fat intake to 10-20gm/day. This can be accomplished by a limited use of meat and dairy products and by using nonfat or lowfat dairy products. Consume organic foods, which are higher in vitamins and minerals and free of pesticides. Beneficial bacteria cultures should be maintained in the gut through increased intake of foods with active cultures or supplementation with probiotics.

GSH: To increase GSH levels, protect against heavy metal toxicity, and increase antioxidant activity, take ALA, the sustained release form, at 300mg/day and NAC at 500mg twice/day on an empty stomach. PS, 300mg/day, is recommended to reduce cortisol and inhibit release of TNF.

Vitamin E (200-600 IU/day), selenium (up to 200mcg/day), and vitamin C (up to 1000mg/day) are important for additional antioxidant supplementation. It is important to use d-alpha tocopherol, the natural form of vitamin E, not dl-alpha tocopherol, which is synthetic. Also, it is essential to use a product that contains mixed tocopherols, the class of molecules constituting vitamin E, which may be as important if not more important than alpha-tocopherol for certain functions in the body.

Vitamin B12: The methylcobalamin form is recommended at 1-2mg/day. This form is available through Thorne Research.

Vitamin D: The average multivitamin contains only small amounts of vitamin D. 4000IU is recommended and is safe based on current scientific evidence.

Melatonin: A small amount of melatonin, between 0.2-1.0mg at bedtime, is suggested.

Antigen-antibody complexes: Supplements that reduce antigen-antibody complexes are pancreatin (350-700mg three times/day between meals using a 10X preparation), bromelain (2400GDU two to four times/day on an empty stomach), and papain (follow product directions). By itself, bromelain may be the best single enzyme to use. There are quite a few combined products that are quite useful. For proper dosing, follow the manufacturer's directions on the label.

Maldigestion and malabsorption: In the presence of symptoms of improper digestion, plant digestive enzymes and nutrient products for gut healing should be considered and are available through Tyler.

Infection: Determine if there is any evidence for infection, such as Chlamydia pneumoniae, and treat appropriately.

Glycine: A daily dose of 7.5gm of threonine, a precursor to glycine, is recommended.

Magnesium: At least 200mg twice/day of magnesium is recommended. To avoid diarrhea, take with 400mg of calcium.

Inosine: To raise uric acid levels, taking up to 5gm/day of inosine, is suggested. Monitor uric acid levels for gout.

Supplements: Due to its safety, the scientific evidence, and our experience with it in practice, a three-month trial of Padma 28, using two tablets three times/day is suggested. Patients have reported the onset of benefit at three months. Padma 28 is available from Econugenics in the U.S. Also to be considered are St. John's Wort (300mg three times/day), taurine (500mg twice/day on an empty stomach), turmeric extract (900mg/day), and two Ayurvedic herbs, Ashwagandha (500mg twice/day) and Bacopa (100mg twice/day with meals). Ginkgo biloba (60mg twice/day) may need to be supplemented under physician supervision as discussed in the herbal supplements section of this chapter.

A multivitamin-mineral supplement: This should be an encapsulated powder, with chelated minerals and free of any type of additive. It should include, among other vitamins and minerals, 10mg of vitamin B6, 150mg of niacin, and 10mg of riboflavin.

Additional modalities: An aerobic exercise practice is recommended in addition to an internal practice such as meditation, imagery, or prayer, which may help emotionally and influence the disease process. Also, there may be a significant therapeutic benefit from acupuncture.

Medications: The appropriate use of medications, including the immune modulating drugs, is to be explored with and supervised by a physician.

Health hazards: Avoid hydrogenated oils, MSG, aspartame, simple sugars, heavy metals (found in some cosmetics, dental fillings, cookware, antacids and antiperspirants with aluminum, and contaminated fish), pesticides in foods, and exposure to pesticides through their use.

Chapter One Supplement Chart

Supplement	Dose	Frequency	Instructions
Alpha-lipoic acid	300mg	Day	Sustained release
Ashwagandha	500mg	Twice/day	
Bacopa	100mg	Twice/day	With meals
Bromelain	2400GDU	Two-four times/day	Empty stomach
Fish oil (DHA & EPA)	500-1000mg	Day	Pesticide and heavy metal free liquid or gel capsules
Ginkgo biloba	60mg	Twice/day	Use with caution with platelet inhibitors or anticoagulants

Supplement	Dose	Frequency	Instructions
GLA & linoleic acid	250mg	Day	
Inosine	Up to 5gm	Day	Monitor uric acid levels for gout
Magnesium	200mg	Twice/day	To avoid diarrhea, may be combined with 400mg calcium
Melatonin	0.2-1mg	Day	Bedtime
N-acetyl cysteine	500mg	Twice/day	Empty stomach
Niacin	150mg	Day	
Padma 28	2 tablets	Three times/day	
Pancreatin	350-700mg	Three times/day	
Phosphatidyl-serine	300mg	Day	
Riboflavin	10mg	Day	
Selenium	200mcg	Day	
St. John's Wort	300mg	Three times/day	
Taurine	500mg	Twice/day	Empty stomach
Threonine	7.5gm	Day	
Turmeric extract	900mg	Day	
Vitamin B12	1-2mg	Day	Use methylcobala-min
Vitamin B6	10mg	Day	

Supplement	Dose	Frequency	Instructions
Vitamin C	Up to 1000mg	Day	
Vitamin D	Up to 4000IU	Day	
Vitamin E	200-600IU	Day	Use d-alpha tocopherol in a mixed tocopherol preparation

Chapter Two

Parkinson's Disease

Parkinson's disease (PD) is a degenerative disorder of the central nervous system (CNS) that affects approximately one million people in the U.S. One in 100 people over fifty-five years of age has PD. Motor symptoms include resting tremor, rigidity, bradykinesia (slowness of movement), gait disorder, and postural instability. Cognitive symptoms include memory impairment, spatial difficulty, impaired processing speed, and occasionally, hallucinations. Pathologically there is degeneration of dopamine neurons in the pars compacta of the substantia nigra, a structure in the midbrain. The diseased cells contain inclusion bodies called Lewy bodies. Neurodegeneration and Lewy bodies are found in other parts of the brain as well. In addition to dopamine systems, PD effects norepinephrine, serotonin, and acetylcholine pathways.[124] The disease progresses over five to fifteen years until there is significant loss of mobility and impaired activities of daily living. The roles of toxicity, free radical damage, inflammation, and mitochondrial dysfunction in PD are becoming clearer. This information lends itself to fairly specific nutritional and herbal treatments directed at detoxification, oxidative adaptation, reduction of inflammation, and mitochondrial protection.

Section 1. Diet and Lifestyle: A number of studies have examined dietary factors in relationship to the occurrence and progression of PD. For example, consuming higher than average levels of carbohydrates, such as sweet foods, has been shown to increase PD risk.[125,126] Before disease onset, patients also have been shown to consume more iron than controls.[127] Increased iron intake as a PD risk factor is supported by research showing higher than normal iron in the substantia nigra of PD patients' brains, which could lead to an increased production of tissue-damaging oxidative radicals (discussed in Section 3).[128] Another factor related to oxidative radicals and PD is vitamin E, a known antioxidant. Men and women with high intake of dietary vitamin E have been shown to have significantly reduced risk of PD.[129] This work was further supported by an examination of plasma levels of vitamin E that showed PD patients had lower vitamin E levels than that of controls.[130] Vitamin E dosage is 200-600 IU/day. It is important to use the d-alpha tocopherol, or natural, form of vitamin E. Also, it is essential to use a product that contains mixed tocopherols, the class of molecules constituting vitamin E, which may be as important if not more important than alpha-tocopherol for certain functions in the body. Inflammation may also play a significant role in PD as suggested by human and animal studies.[131,132] Further evidence for the role of inflammation in PD comes from promising results with different anti-inflammatory treatments in several animal models of PD.[133] Inflammation is discussed in general in the introductory chapter and is discussed specifically regarding PD in Section 8 of this chapter. Pesticide and heavy metal exposure have also been shown to increase PD risk and these topics are further discussed below (Section 2).

Bowel health often can be improved by adding fiber to the diet. Plant cell walls contain about 35% water insoluble fibers such as cellulose and 45% water-soluble fibers such as hemicelluloses, mucilages, gums, and pectins. Insoluble fiber binds water, which increases fecal size and weight, thus reducing constipation, a common problem in PD. Astarloa, et al. studied the effects of a diet rich in insoluble fiber in PD patients on Sinemet (L-dopa).[134] This diet reduced constipation, increased L-dopa absorption with higher plasma concentration, and improved motor function. This study suggests that insoluble fiber, such as wheat bran and ground flax seed, be added to the PD patient's diet.

Large neutral amino acids compete with L-dopa for the same carrier system across the blood-brain barrier. Studies show that increased large neutral amino acids in the blood decrease mobility and on-time in patients on L-dopa. This is the basis for the recommendation of a decreased protein diet (0.75-0.8g/kg-body weight/day) and for a protein redistribution diet. The redistribution allows for 10% of the protein during daytime and the remainder in the evening. This diet should be used cautiously because of the risk of a negative nitrogen balance, or a breakdown of tissue protein and the possibility of diminished mineral and vitamin intake.[135] Berry, et al. studied various carbohydrate:protein ratio diets in terms of symptomatology in PD patients on L-dopa. They found a 5:1 carbohydrate:protein diet proved superior to other diets in terms of motor performance.[136]

Section 2. Toxic Exposure: Humans are exposed to a large variety of toxins (xenobiotics) including food components, environmental toxins, and pharmaceuticals. We have complex enzyme systems in the liver to detoxify these substances. These systems vary from individual to individual depending upon genetics, lifestyle, and environment. Although some studies are contradictory, there is a general consensus that the ability to detoxify and eliminate these substances affects the onset and course of PD. Patients with familial and nonfamilial PD have been shown to have liver enzyme genes associated with poor liver function.[137,138] A diminished ability for the liver to remove neurotoxins such as pesticides could increase the risk of PD.[139] The reason PD risk increases with age may be the reduced ability of the aging liver to detoxify, which would result in increased levels of xenobiotics remaining in the bloodstream.[140]

Epidemiological and experimental data suggest an increased risk of PD in individuals exposed to neurotoxicants such as herbicides and pesticides.[141,142,143,144,145,146,147,148,149,150] The results of a California study showed a dose-response for insecticide use[151] and another study showed a dose-response relation between PD risk and lifetime exposure to field crop farming and to grain farming.[152] Pesticides are also directly toxic to mitochondria, which have been shown to be dysfunctional in PD patients (see Section 6).[153] Very telling is a postmortem study of twenty PD patients by Fleming, et al. in Florida. Pesticide residues were assayed in twenty PD brains, seven brains with AD and fourteen non-neurological controls. Dieldren, an organochlorine pesticide for locust control was found in six of twenty PD brains, one of seven AD brains, and in none of the controls. Dieldren is a lipid soluble, long-lasting mitochondrial poison and may well play a role in PD given the mitochondrial defects in this disorder.[154] DDT was found in a majority of the PD, AD, and control brains, confirming the widespread human exposure to environmental chemicals. Susceptibility to the effects of pesticides and other xenobiotics may depend on variability in toxin metabolism related to differences found in PD patient liver enzyme genes compared to those of controls. One study examining several xenobiotics found a similar increase in PD risk among people who used cleaning supplies in their work.[155] Of interest is that cigarette smoking appears to reduce the PD risk. This is thought to be related to the increase in certain detoxification enzymes (cytochrome P450) in smokers due to the polyaromatic hydrocarbons in tobacco smoke. However, the serious risks of smoking far outweigh this protective benefit.

Heavy metal intoxication is a serious issue in the U.S. with estimates of 25% of the population having significant heavy metal toxicity.[156] Sources of toxicity are numerous including mercury toxicity from silver dental amalgam.[157] A study in Singapore examined mercury intake by looking at fish consumption, ethnic over-the-counter medication use, occupational exposure and possession of dental amalgam fillings. They found a monotonic dose-response association between PD and blood mercury levels. Blood and urine were good predictors of PD but hair levels were not.[158] A multi-center study in Germany found more frequent exposure to heavy metals, and a larger number of amalgam-filled teeth, in PD patients than in controls.[159] Gorell, et al. found a significant association of PD in individuals in the Detroit area with more than a twenty-year exposure to copper and manganese. There was a stronger correlation of PD with more than twenty years exposure to lead-copper, lead-iron and iron-copper than to any one metal alone. Their conclusion is that " … chronic exposure to these metals is associated with PD, and that they may act alone or together over time to help produce the disease."[160] The overloading of brain tissue with heavy metals also may worsen PD neurodegeneration by triggering inflammatory processes.[161]

It should be added that much progress in PD research stemmed from studies on 1-methyl-4-phenyl-1,2,3,6-tetrahydropyridine (MPTP), a designer heroin-like drug that resulted in very rapid onset PD in the individuals using it. Not only did the discoveries around MPTP strengthen concerns regarding xenobiotic toxicity but its mechanism of injury served as a template for understanding the role of glutamate and the mitochondria in PD. MPTP is converted to the active neurotoxic agent MPP(+) by astrocytes, cells that provide structural and physiological support to neurons. In turn, MPP(+) impairs astrocyte metabolism and reduces glutamate reuptake. This results in an increase of extracellular glutamate, which is an excitotoxic neurotransmitter.[162] In addition, MPP(+) inhibits complex I of the mitochondrial electron transport chain and increases free radical production.[163] All these changes result in a cascade of events ending in programmed cell death (apoptosis).

PD patients in general should strengthen their bodies' detoxification abilities with high potency vitamin/mineral supplements. Unless anemia is present, iron should be avoided as well as copper in the vitamin/mineral supplement. In particular, one should emphasize minerals like calcium, magnesium, zinc, and chromium- and sulfur-containing amino acids (methionine, cysteine, and taurine), and high sulfur containing foods such as garlic, onions, and eggs. In addition, water-soluble fibers including guar gum, oat bran, pectin, psyllium seed, and ground flax seed are helpful. It is important to note that organic produce is not only significantly higher in vitamins and minerals but also lower in heavy metals and herbicides. For these reasons, organic produce is strongly recommended. In PD patients with known toxin exposure, the use of liver supportive herbs appears to be indicated to help reduce any ongoing toxicity contributing to progression of the disease. The primary hepatic protective herb is milk thistle, either as a liquid extract or a solid, standardized extract, at 175mg twice/day. Two other liver herbs, turmeric (900mg/day) and schizandra (500-1000mg/day) may actually have a more specific effect on increasing the liver's detoxifying ability. Schizandra probably is best used when there is toxic exposure or some type of acute illness involving fatigue or respiratory involvement. We have not recommended it clinically for long-term use in PD. A blended extract with multiple liver herbs probably would be superior to taking one herb alone.

A full detoxification program is more complex and requires a complete evaluation of the individual. Hair and urine analysis for heavy metals may be helpful, although a more sensitive measure of body burden requires an oral or intravenous challenge with a heavy metal chelator, 2,3-dimercapto-1-propanesulfonic acid (DMPS). Mercury is tightly bound in the body to molecular species called sulfhydryl groups and may not be excreted enough to be detected on standard heavy metal assays of hair or urine. Another substance, 2,3-dimercaptosuccinic acid (DMSA), also can be given IV or by mouth for detection of increased body burdens of heavy metals. If toxic levels of heavy metals are found, then treatment by someone experienced with detoxification and the issues surrounding the central nervous system (CNS), liver, and kidney is recommended.

Section 3. Oxidative stress: Oxidation, the deterioration of tissue caused by specific chemical reactions involving oxygen, can occur with exposure to environmental toxins or chemical food additives, or as the result of normal metabolism. Adenosine triphosphate (ATP) carries cellular energy and is generated via the electron transport chain in mitochondria. Its production is associated with free radical formation, molecules containing unpaired electrons in orbitals that attack other molecular species for electrons, causing oxidation. Free radicals are generated by numerous other reactions including the formation of uric acid via xanthine oxidase, intoxication by heavy metals and the metabolism of xenobiotic chemicals.[164] Free radicals serve important biologic functions including their use by phagocytic white blood cells to destroy bacteria and other foreign matter and cells. However, they are also dangerous molecular species and the body has an antioxidant molecular system to contain their activity. Free radicals, including hydrogen peroxide, superoxide anion, and the hydroxyl radical, will attack and destroy the structural integrity of lipids, proteins, and DNA. Of interest is that the metabolism of dopamine itself creates free radicals including hydrogen peroxide and the hydroxyl radical. It also appears that environmental neurotoxins ultimately act via oxidative stress.[165]

There is evidence of increased oxidation in the substantia nigra of PD brains with increased lipid peroxidation (oxidized lipids) and decreased reduced-glutathione. Glutathione (GSH) is an essential intracellular antioxidant that needs to be in a reduced state to be effective. The enzymes involved in antioxidant defense, glutathione peroxidase (GP) and catalase, are diminished in PD as well. It is well known that the presence of iron can increase oxidative reactions. Total iron is increased in the substantia nigra in PD patients compared to individuals without PD, and neuromelanin, resulting from the auto-oxidation of dopamine, serves as a reservoir for iron in the substantia nigra.[166] Unfortunately, as the disease progresses, there is increased metabolism of dopamine resulting in increased free radical formation.

The evidence for oxidative damage in PD recommends the use of antioxidants. A study by S. Fahn at Columbia University in 1992 found that the combined use of high dose vitamins C and E increased the time until L-dopa was needed in PD patients by 2.5 years.[167] Three antioxidants that may prove very important in PD are alpha-lipoic acid (ALA), GSH, and N-acetyl cysteine (NAC). ALA is a low molecular weight substance absorbed from the diet that crosses the blood-brain barrier. It is reduced in cells to dihydrolipoate, which is partially exported to the extracellular medium.

Through improvement in brain metabolic function, ALA may provide neuroprotective effects.[168] It may be the premier antioxidant for the CNS because it is both water and fat soluble, exists in both the intra and extracellular space, is involved, through redox cycling, in the regeneration of other antioxidants like vitamins C and E, and it increases GSH levels. ALA also is a chelator for ferrous iron, copper, and cadmium, helping to keep these metals in their appropriate cellular compartments. ALA can be taken in sustained release form, 300mg/day.

GSH, one of the main intracellular antioxidants, is deficient in PD patients and the magnitude of reduction parallels the severity of the disease.[169] GSH maintains vitamins E and C in their reduced state and removes potentially damaging peroxides. It is not well absorbed when taken orally but can be administered IV. A 1996 study in Italy found significant improvement in PD patients given 600mg GSH IV twice/day. There was a 42% decline in overall disability using two different rating scales and the therapeutic effect lasted 2-4 months after cessation of IV therapy.[170] IV GSH treatment may be considered and obtained from an MD with a holistic or integrated practice.

NAC, an endogenous antioxidant, also helps in detoxifying the body of heavy metals such as mercury and lead, environmental pollutants, and certain pesticides. It increases intracellular cysteine levels, which leads to increased GSH concentrations, and inhibits nitric oxide production. Its daily dosage is 500mg twice/day on an empty stomach.[171] NAC also reduces the deposition of an abnormal protein called alpha-synuclein. This subject will be discussed at some length later in the chapter.

Other compounds of interest in antioxidant adaptation include melatonin and the herb milk thistle. Melatonin is a free radical scavenger, which means it removes free radicals, and stimulates gene expression for antioxidant enzymes including GP, copper-zinc dismutase, and manganese superoxide dismutase.[172] A common dosage for melatonin is 1mg at bedtime. Milk thistle inhibits xanthine oxidase, the enzyme that converts xanthine to uric acid plus superoxide radical.[173] The alternate pathway, xanthine dehydrogenase, which converts xanthine to uric acid plus nicotinamide adenine dinucleotide (NADH), is preferable because it does not result in superoxide radical production. Milk thistle dosage is 175mg twice/day.

Section 4. Dopamine: With progression of PD there are decreased amounts of dopamine. The rate-limiting step in synthesis of dopamine from tyrosine involves tyrosine hydroxylase. NADH supplies reducing equivalents as a coenzyme in this reaction. NADH appears to increase dopamine production in tissue cultures and in humans, and IV and oral administration of NADH improves performance on PD rating scales.[174] In 1993 in Vienna, a trial with oral NADH in 885 PD patients was conducted. 80% of the patients showed a mildly beneficial response with 19.3% having a more significant response. Younger patients or those with a shorter duration of illness showed a more marked improvement with NADH.[175] In addition, the repair of oxidative damage to DNA requires high levels of NADH. Dosage for NADH is 5mg twice/day. It is also of note that the B vitamin nicotinamide, a precursor of NADH, acts as a free radical scavenger and is able to block the destruction of neurons caused by the designer street drug MPTP. These actions make nicotinamide (500mg twice/day) of interest in PD.[176]

Mucuna Pruriens (velvet beans) is an Ayurvedic herb with a high concentration of L-dopa. Solaray has a product, DopaBean, which is mucuna pruriens. Each capsule contains

50mg of L-dopa. The advantage of an herbal form of L-dopa is the antioxidant properties of the additional constituents in the preparation. On the other hand, the lack of carbidopa may reduce the amount of L-dopa available for transport into the CNS. Addition of carbidopa, by itself, is a consideration. The DopaBean dosage would depend upon the individual's response to the herb but the equivalent dosage of L-dopa in the mucana pruriens to the patient's current pharmaceutical dosage of L-dopa is a reasonable goal.

Dopaminergic medications can cause extensive side effects including mood changes and sleep difficulties thought to be related to reduced levels of 5-hydroxytryptophan (5HTP), an immediate precursor of serotonin. In patients taking L-dopa, 5HTP can counteract the side effects on mood and sleep and also improve physical symptoms.[177] In patients not on L-dopa, 5HTP may worsen symptoms, particularly rigidity.

Section 5. Excitotoxicity: The neurotransmitter glutamate may play a role in PD. PD patients have decreased oxidative phosphorylation in the mitochondria, which results in impaired energy production and a drop in the transmembrane potential. This drop in potential reduces the magnesium blockade of the N-methyl-D-aspartate (NMDA) receptor on the cell surface. Glutamate stimulates the NMDA receptor, and if the magnesium blockade is reduced, a calcium influx into the cell results. This influx of calcium initiates a cascade of events including activation of nitric oxide synthase with increased nitric oxide production. In addition, there is increased free radical production and activation of proteases and lipases. Increased intracellular calcium also favors the xanthine oxidase pathway to uric acid over the xanthine dehydrogenase pathway. As noted above, the xanthine oxidase pathway to uric acid produces the superoxide radical. Nitric oxide and the superoxide radical combine to form the highly dangerous free radical peroxynitrite, which is involved in a number of damaging cellular events possibly leading to apoptosis.[178] In summary, the essential excitatory neurotransmitter glutamate takes on a dangerous aspect in PD patients. Their reduced cellular energy metabolism can make the excitation from glutamate damaging, and in some circumstances, fatal to the nerve cell being stimulated.

Reducing the damaging effects of excitotoxicity is important, particularly in PD patients. Aspartame[179,180] and MSG, which may increase glutamate levels, should be avoided. The branched chain amino acids L-leucine, L-isoleucine and L-valine increase the conversion of glutamate to the non-excitotoxic amino acid glutamine.[181,182] Because PD patients have reduced spinal fluid levels of branched chain amino acids,[183] it may be advisable to increase the intake of these amino acids with specialized protein supplements such as Spectrum Shake by Nutribiotic or dietary changes such as increased brown rice consumption. The amino acid arginine is metabolized to nitric oxide and citrulline. By increasing citrulline intake, such as in watermelon, the reaction forming nitric oxide may be partially reversed decreasing nitric oxide levels. Finally, the Chinese herb Huperzine A, an acetylcholinesterase inhibitor, also inhibits glutamate stimulation of the NMDA receptor.[184,185] Huperzine A dosage is 50-200mcg twice/day. It is important to note that Viagra should be avoided in PD because it works by increasing nitric oxide production.

Taurine appears to provide significant protection against excitotoxicity. It is a small molecule, related to the amino acids but lacking the carboxyl or acid component. Rather than being a component of proteins, it occurs in free form in the body, manufactured from the amino acid cysteine and vitamin

B6. Numerous scientific studies suggest a role in reducing hypertension, limiting the long-term damage in diabetes and, in general, reducing oxidative stress in the body. Of interest is that the spinal fluid levels of taurine are reduced in PD.[186]

Taurine appears to modulate excitoxicity favorably in multiple ways. It increases the expression of an enzyme, glutamic acid decarboxylase (GAD), responsible for the formation of Gamma-aminobutyric acid (GABA), an important inhibitory and protective neurotransmitter in the nervous system[187] and may directly activate GABA receptors.[188] It also appears to reduce the magnitude of intracellular calcium influx secondary to glutamate excitotoxicity.[189,190] For those readers wishing to understand more about the importance of glutamate, calcium regulation, and excitotoxicity, Dr. Russell Blaylock's book *Excitotoxins: The Taste That Kills* is a scholarly, seminal, yet accessible work on the dangers of excitotoxins, such as MSG and aspartame, in our food.[191] In particular, he outlines a semi-unified theory of neurodegenerative disorders related to glutamate, the essential but potentially harmful excitatory neurotransmitter in our bodies. One of many effects of glutamate is the increase in intracellular calcium. This in turn reduces the energetic power of the mitochondria, the energy furnaces of our cells, and can lead, through second messengers such as protein kinases, to apoptosis. We will also explore in the chapter on AD how taurine appears to block the neurotoxicity of beta-amyloid, the amorphous extracellular protein that plays a role in the development of AD.[192] Because of its multiple beneficial effects, taurine is recommended in PD. The dosage is 500mg twice/day on an empty stomach.

Magnesium is involved in many metabolic reactions including the protection of cells against the deleterious effects of glutamate. Our foods are depleted of magnesium, as they are of many other vitamins and minerals due to the significant loss of nutrient containing topsoil. In addition, fruits and vegetables are picked before they are ripe, before the nutrients have reached their highest levels. Also, the chemicals used in non-organic farming may block the full production of nutrients in the food. As a result, Americans tend to be deficient in magnesium. Supplementation with magnesium, 200mg twice/day is recommended. Also of note is that the PD drug Eldepryl (deprenyl) protects neurons from damage due to glutamate.

Section 6. Mitochondria: Mitochondria extract energy from food nutrients and are the powerhouses of cells. They are found in protozoa, yeast, plants, and animals and contain the enzymes of the Krebs cycle and oxidative phosphorylation (electron transport chain). Mitochondrial enzymes are coded by DNA within the mitochondria itself, derived from the mother. In fact, analysis of mitochondrial DNA reveals the origin of our species 150,000 years ago in Africa. We migrated from Africa into Asia about 60,000 to 70,000 years ago and into Europe about 40,000 to 50,000 years ago.[193] Oxidative damage to DNA, both nuclear and mitochondrial is currently considered a major cause of aging and degenerative disease. Mitochondrial DNA is oxidized at ten times the rate of nuclear DNA. In people over the age of seventy, it is oxidized fifteen times the nuclear DNA rate. This is due to the presence of oxidative phosphorylation in the mitochondria, and the lack of repair mechanisms and protective proteins (histones).[194]

In the 1980s, the designer street drug MPTP caused severe PD in its users and drew attention to the role of the mitochondria in PD. MPTP inhibits NADH dehydrogenase, an early step in the electron transport chain in mitochondria. This inhibition increases the concentration of the superoxide radical, hydrogen peroxide, and the hydroxyl radical, which are associated with destruction of DNA.[195] MPP(+), the active metabolite of MPTP, also reduces cellular levels of GSH, a cardinal intracellular antioxidant. This phenomenon may be secondary to reduced mitochondrial energy production in the presence of MPP(+).[196] The mechanism of injury by MPTP has been very helpful in understanding what may happen in the natural occurrence of PD. For example, toxins in the environment (xenobiotics) may injure the mitochondria in PD patients in a manner similar to the toxic effects of MPTP.

PD patients have a significant reduction in complex I (NADH:ubiquinone oxidoreductase) activity of the mitochondrial electron transport chain in multiple tissues including platelets. Ubiquinone is another name for Coenzyme Q10 (CoQ10). Recent genetic studies suggest that this defect in complex I may arise from point mutations in mitochondrial DNA.[197] There is also evidence that chronic administration of levodopa can alter mitochondrial respiratory chain activity in rats, a finding supporting the position that chronic L-dopa administration may contribute to progression of PD.[198] This latter article also reported that vitamin C and deprenyl prevent the inhibitory effect of levodopa and dopamine on complex I activity. Our findings support the use of antioxidants and monoamine oxidase (MAO) inhibitors as therapeutic strategies in attempts to slow the progression of PD. Monoamine oxidase is one of several enzymes that breaks down dopamine after it communicates between nerve cells. The medication deprenyl is an MAO inhibitor used in PD. Another enzyme that breaks down dopamine is Catechol-o-methyl transferase (COMT). An inhibitor of this is the medication Comtan. Deprenyl may not provide much symptomatic relief but, as noted above, may have long-term benefits in PD. Comtan, on the other hand, actively prolongs a single dose of L-dopa and has immediate therapeutic benefits.

A number of studies in animals and humans have demonstrated that oral supplementation with CoQ10 increases complex I activity.[199] Supplementation with CoQ10 also appears to protect neurons against neurotoxic agents. Repleting the known CoQ10 deficiency in PD would increase mitochondrial energy production, reduce free radical formation, improve cellular membrane potential, and thereby protect against excitotoxic stimulation and xenobiotic injury (xenobiotics act in part through oxidative damage). A recent study organized through the University of California, San Diego demonstrated that supplementation with 1200mg/day of CoQ10 resulted in significantly less disability for a treated group of individuals compared with a control group over a sixteen-month interval of time.[200] Less benefit was seen for 300mg/day and 600mg/day. This work is further supported by PD clinical research showing promising effects and symptomatic benefit from CoQ10.[201,202] Another recent study also demonstrated that CoQ10 could slow the progression of PD.[203] CoQ10 appears to be an important supplement for PD patients. Although the traditional dosage is 100-200mg/day, the recent University of California, San Diego study suggests 1200mg/day, preferably in three-four divided doses with food.

Ginkgo biloba, a possible monoamine oxidase inhibitor,[204] would also ameliorate the inhibiting effect of monoamine metabolites on complex I activity, perhaps in part by inhibiting the free radical production involved in the metabolism of dopamine. Dosage is 40mg Ginkgo biloba three times/day or 60mg twice/day. Ginkgo biloba needs to be supplemented carefully when other platelet inhibitors or anticoagulants are being used. This includes the supplements vitamin E and essential fatty acids and the drugs Coumadin, aspirin, Ticlid, and Aggrenox. In the presence of heart disease or stroke, or when an individual is on numerous medications, physician supervision should be available when using Ginkgo biloba.

Section 7. Alpha-synuclein: Alpha-synuclein is a protein found in nerve cells everywhere in the brain. It is particularly enriched in presynaptic terminals, the tips of nerve cell branches that make contact, in structures called synapses, with other nerve cells. The function of alpha-synuclein in the brain is only recently being elucidated. Its enrichment in nerve terminals suggests a role in synapse maintenance and plasticity.[205] Plasticity is the name for structural and biochemical changes made by neurons in response to demands placed on the brain. Every nerve cell has numerous synapses with other nerve cells and the plasticity of this dense forest of connections acts as a record of our individual human experience. Other possible roles of alpha-synuclein involve participation in signaling pathways, cell differentiation, cell survival, and dopamine neurotransmission.[206]

Alpha-synuclein appears to be involved in neurodegenerative disorders. It was initially found, in fragmented form, in the senile amyloid plaques of AD. Subsequently, two mutations were discovered in the gene responsible for alpha-synuclein in genetic (autosomal dominant) PD. Autosomal dominant PD accounts for only a small fraction of cases. Ultimately, alpha-synuclein was found to be a major constituent of Lewy bodies, the signature pathological abnormality in common PD. This protein then appears involved in both the development of AD and PD. It is also found in amyotrophic lateral sclerosis (Lou Gehrig's disease) and a disorder called multiple system atrophy.

Although its role in these diseases is not clear, it is known that under normal circumstances, the alpha-synuclein protein is usually unfolded in a shape called the alpha helical form. Various factors, including the gene mutations noted above, and probably oxidative stress, causes the protein to assume a beta-folded shape.[207] This shape is prone to aggregate with other beta-folded molecules assuming insoluble fibrils in the brain. A recent Parkinsonism model has proven that several pesticides can also stimulate the formation of alpha-synuclein fibrils.[208] This change in the protein would result in loss of its function, contributing in some manner to the disease process, such as formation of Lewy bodies found in PD.

A study at University of California, San Diego studied alpha-synuclein's sensitivity to oxidative stress. Placing the protein under oxidative stress resulted in the abnormal aggregation of the protein. Of interest is that the process could be blocked by NAC, an important antioxidant supplement.[209] This is another rationale for supplementation of NAC (500mg twice/day on an empty stomach) in PD.

Section 8. Inflammation: The Introduction contains a general discussion of inflammation, all of which is relevant to PD. Below is a discussion of additional PD specific aspects of inflammation. There is increasing evidence that inflammation plays a significant role in PD. The CNS has its own unique inflammatory cells called microglia, which are ubiquitous throughout the CNS and help to maintain neuronal health. It has been known since 1988 that microglia are activated in the abnormal parts of the PD brain, namely the substantia nigra and the basal ganglia. The microglia secrete proinflammatory substances that are increased in the spinal fluid and brain of PD patients.[210,211] These mediators, called cytokines, include tumor necrosis factor-alpha (TNF-α), interleukin (IL)-1beta, IL-2, IL-4, and IL-6.[212] Two enzymes related to inflammation, nitric oxide synthase and nicotinamide adenine dinucleotide phosphate-reduced (NADPH) oxidase are also induced in PD. The first enzyme creates nitric oxide, which can activate a cascade of enzymes leading to apoptosis.[213] The latter enzyme leads to molecules called reactive oxygen species (ROS) and a number of other chemicals toxic to nerve cells. ROS activate microglia, causing a self-reinforcing cycle, since microglia generate the NADPH oxidase that in turn generates ROS. Activated microglia, in addition to secreting proinflammatory substances, secrete an excitotoxin called quinolinic acid.

An excitotoxin is a substance, either intrinsic to the body's chemistry or coming from outside the body, that excites nerve cells. In excess, excitotoxins injure nerve cells and initiate a cascade of chemical events leading to cell death (apoptosis). The injury caused by intrinsic excitotoxins such as quinolinic acid is intimately related to the inflammatory process discussed above. Other potential excitotoxins in the body include the neurotransmitter glutamate (related to MSG used as a flavor enhancer) and the amino acid homocysteine, a known risk factor for heart disease, stroke, and AD. Both glutamate and homocysteine are intimately related to the inflammatory process.[214,215,216,217] In fact, the enzyme responsible for production of nitric oxide is tightly coupled to an enzyme associated with inflammation, Cyclooxygenase-2 (COX-2), in excitotoxic nerve cell injury.[218] In addition, homocysteine up-regulates or activates nuclear factor kappaB, an intracellular signaling molecule for inflammation discussed below.

COX-2 and 5-lipooxygenase (5-LOX), enzymes that are significant components of inflammation, are also expressed by activated microglia. COX-2, present in the body only during inflammatory states, converts arachidonic acid into inflammatory molecules called prostaglandins, whereas 5-LOX converts arachidonic acid into inflammatory molecules called leukotrienes. Prostaglandins and leukotrienes are called eicosanoids and can be powerful and potentially harmful to the body. It is important to note that inhibitors of the COX-2 and 5-LOX pathways protect nerve cells from injury.[219] The new class of anti-inflammatory drugs including Celebrex, Vioxx, and Bextra inhibit primarily COX-2. These anti-inflammatories were thought to have fewer side effects than drugs such as Motrin, Naprosyn, and Tolectin, which inhibit both Cyclooxygenase-1 (COX-1) and COX-2, thereby reducing the protective effects of prostaglandins on the stomach and kidney. Clinical studies over the last five to ten years cast doubt on their increased safety, particularly in regards to potential effects on the heart.

Nutrients and herbs that inhibit PD inflammatory processes should be part of the supplemental protocol for PD patients. Because of the complexity of inflammation, herbs, and nutrients that interrupt as many of the components of the inflammatory cascades as possible are preferred. Bromelain has multiple anti-inflammatory effects and is quite safe to use. Dosage is up to 2400GDU four times/day. There are at least nine plants that have shown COX-2 inhibition. These are baikal skullcap, turmeric, feverfew, ginger, green tea, holy basil, nettle leaf, oregano, and rosemary.[220] An extract, Nexrutine (250mg/day), derived from the bark of the phellodendron tree of Asia also is a COX-2 inhibitor. Although possibly not as prevalent, natural inhibitors of 5-LOX include extracts of the Ayurvedic herb Boswellia,[221] extracts of the Chinese medicinal herb Atractylodes,[222] and turmeric.[223] Selection and dosage of these herbs would depend upon the personal preference of the patient as well as the presence of other medical conditions.

Turmeric may be the best and safest anti-inflammatory to add to the supplemental regimen in PD. Not only does it inhibit both COX-2 and 5-LOX enzymes, it appears to suppress the effects of TNF,[224] another powerful mediator in inflammation and apoptosis, and to inhibit Nuclear factor-kappa B (NF-kappa B) activation.[225] NF-kappa B is an intracellular signaling molecule. Microglia manufacture COX-2, as well as other proinflammatory substances, in response to NF-kappa B. This single molecule plays a role in a wide variety of processes in the body including inflammation, immunity, cancer, and apoptosis.[226,227] Regulating NF-kappa B would be a particularly powerful way to control a number of pathological processes including inflammation. This is called upstream modulation of inflammation versus controlling the downstream enzymes such as COX-2 and 5-LOX. In herbology, turmeric has a number of other uses including use as a liver tonic and in ulcer disease. For the older PD patient on a number of other medicines, including aspirin and standard anti-inflammatory agents, turmeric can be protective in this setting. A common dosage of a turmeric extract is 900mg/day.

The omega-3 fatty acids, docosahexaenoic acid (DHA) and eicosapentaenoic acid (EPA), can reduce inflammation, especially in combination with omega-6 fatty acids. Omega-3 and -6 fatty acids are discussed at length in the chapter on MS. DHA and EPA are found in fish oil. Dosage is approximately 500-1000mg/day of DHA plus EPA and can be taken in gel-capsule form. It is important to take oil from fish that lived in unpolluted waters free from heavy metals and pesticide residues. The label on the bottle should make reference to assays showing no heavy metals or various pesticide residues. Carlson's Norwegian Cod Liver Oil and Nordic Naturals provide such products. Gamma linoleic acid (GLA) is an omega-6 fatty acid found in borage oil, black currant seed oil, and evening primrose oil. Dosage for omega-6 fatty acids is 250-500mg/day of GLA plus linoleic acid. A study in 2003 at the Harvard School of Public Health found that several markers of inflammation, including TNF and C-reactive protein, were proportionately reduced as subjects increased their intake of omega-3 fatty acids. This was seen for DHA and EPA, the main fatty acids in fish oil, but not for alpha linolenic and cis-linoleic acids found in flaxseed oil. Of interest also is that intake of omega-6 fatty acids increased the anti-inflammatory effect of the omega-3 fatty acids.[228]

It is established that sugar intake increases the inflammatory process. A 2004 study at the University of New York at Buffalo revealed that healthy individuals had increases of free radicals as well as NF-kappa B following ingestion of a glucose solution.[229] This suggests that sugar may increase the inflammatory cascade both upstream and downstream. Patients with PD would be well advised to avoid simple sugars such as that found in most candy, sodas, and many sweet foods.

Section 9. Ubiquitin-proteasomal (UPS) system: In the last few years, there have been several major discoveries that may have a significant impact on our ability to prevent the onset and mitigate the progression of the neurological disorders discussed in this book. The 2004 Nobel Prize was given to three scientists, Aaron Ciechanover, Aram Hershko, and Irwin Rose for advancing our understanding of the breakdown of proteins in our cells. In order to maintain an equilibrium, or homeostasis, of the amount of cellular proteins, including enzymes, signaling molecules, and structural components, formation of proteins needs to be balanced with protein degradation. In addition, oxidized, aggregated, or misfolded proteins need to be identified and metabolized. The most important protein-degrading, or proteolytic, system in every cell is the ubiquitin-proteasomal system, the understanding of which resulted in the Nobel Prize noted above. There is increasing evidence that dysfunction of this system plays a particular role in PD and AD and may play a role in stroke and MS.

The UPS consists of ubiquitin (a protein) and the proteasome (a complex multi-protein structure). In simple terms, ubiquitin attaches to the protein to be digested, presenting the protein to the barrel-shaped proteasome for digestion. Ubiquitin is actually a cascade of three successive enzymes that attach to the target protein. The identified protein is then digested inside the cylindrically shaped proteasome consisting of a core (20S) enzymatic (protease) unit with two (19S) regulatory particles (also called the PA700 proteasome activator).

Proteasomal activity decreases with aging. In the brain, this occurs in the cortex as well as in deeper structures, including the basal ganglia, large subcortical gray matter structures involved in movement. In one study of rats, this decline was found in the cerebral cortex and hippocampus but was not seen in the brain stem or cerebellum,[230] while another study of rats, mice, and marmosets suggested particular reduction with age in the striatum, globus pallidus, and substantia nigra regions involved in PD.[231] Since the proteasome metabolizes oxidized proteins and prevents protein aggregation, loss of function with age suggests a role in PD and AD, in which protein oxidation and aggregation play important roles. It also is known that the function of mitochondria, the main intracellular organelles responsible for energy production, declines with aging as well as in neurodegenerative disorders. A study in 2004 at the University of Kentucky demonstrated that inhibition of proteasome function results in dramatically reduced function of complex I and II in the mitochondrial electron transport chain.[232] This study suggests that a decline in proteasomal function may play a role in the loss mitochondrial function, and hence cellular energy, with aging.

Starting in about 2000, multiple research centers in the US and abroad have demonstrated diminished proteasomal function in AD. As noted in the chapter on AD, the brain in this disorder reveals intracellular neurofibrillary tangles (paired helical filaments – PHFs) and extracellular beta-amyloid plaques. A recent study from Berlin demonstrated a decrease of proteasomal function to 56% of normal in a sample of AD cortex. It also appeared that the PHFs were bound to proteasomes and the degree of binding correlated with the amount of functional loss of proteasomal activity. A separate part of the study revealed that the PHF tau protein inhibited the proteasome to the point where the cell would degenerate and die.[233] Of interest is that PHFs consist of an insoluble aggregation of normally soluble tau protein. AD then seems to involve a positive feedback system in which an early inability of the proteasome to prevent tau aggregation results in PHFs that induce further loss of function of the proteasome. Why then does this not occur in all aging brains? Since the UPS genetics are complex, it may be possible that a certain genetic makeup accelerates this self-inducing process resulting in clinical AD.

The relationship between UPS and PD is more complex and in some ways more explanatory of the origin of PD. In 2001, researchers in England demonstrated for the first time a significant drop in proteasome function in the substantia nigra, the black substance in the brainstem containing dopamine neurons that die in PD.[234] It also was discovered that Lewy bodies, the intracytoplasmic inclusions characteristic of PD contain the aggregated proteins of alpha-synuclein as well as ubiquitin the signaling protein of the UPS. In addition, it has been demonstrated in PD that aggregated alpha-synuclein binds and potently inhibits the proteasome similar to the effect of paired helical filaments in AD.[235] Another interesting observation is that several genetic mutations responsible for familial PD code for enzymes playing important roles in the UPS. The enzymes are called Parkin and ubiquitin C-termimal hydrolase L1. Abnormalities in these enzymes degrade the UPS and result in genetically transmitted PD. In summary, loss of function of the UPS appears to play a central role in the development of PD. The process is certainly complex, involving as well, external toxins, oxidative injury, mitochondrial dysfunction and genetic factors.

The role of the UPS in stroke and MS is quite different than its compromised role in the neurodegenerative disorders. The proteasome appears to play an important role in degrading proteins involved in inflammation, cell cycles, growth of new blood vessels (angiogenesis), apoptosis and gene expression. In particular, the UPS system degrades a protein called IkappaB which inhibits NF-kappa B. NF-kappa B is a gene transcription factor that upregulates production of proteins involved in inflammation and cell growth. By degrading IkappaB, the UPS upregulates NF-kappa B resulting in increased inflammation and cell growth. In fact, Velcade (bortezomib) is a new drug approved for use in multiple myeloma. It is thought to inhibit myeloma cells by inhibition of NF-kappa B through its reversible inhibition of the proteasome. Although chronic inflammation plays a role in PD and AD, acute inflammation is more salient in stroke and MS. In regards to stroke, pretreatment of experimental animals with proteasome inhibitors reduces stroke volume and acute degeneration of astrocytes and neurons. In addition, proteasome inhibitors in this animal stroke model suppresses activation of NF-kappa B, presumably by decreasing the degradation of the NF-kappa B inhibitor, IkappaB. The benefit of UPS inhibitors in stroke appears to relate, at least in part, to decreased activity of NF-kappa B.[236] Similarly, in MS, inhibition of inflammation via downregulation of the proteasome is a promising mode of therapy. A study in France in 2001 demonstrated that ritonavir, an HIV-1 protease inhibitor that modulates proteasomal function, inhibited experimental allergic encephalomyelitis in experimental animals.[237] There are no completed trials yet using proteasomal inhibitors in clinical MS.

There is a naturally occurring substance in grapes, peanuts, and pine trees called resveratrol that enhances proteasomal function. Resveratrol, a polyphenol, is an antioxidant compound that helps explain the French paradox. The French paradox is the name for the puzzle as to why many French people eat a high fat diet and yet have reduced rates of heart disease. There are now numerous studies on the health promoting properties of resveratrol, only a fraction of which relate to the French paradox. It is antioxidant,[238] inhibits formation of pro-inflammatory substances, inhibits platelet aggregation, and induces apoptosis in cancer cells.[239] Its anticancer properties are undergoing a number of studies for potential clinical application.[240,241] Resveratrol also reduces nitric oxide levels with consequent reduction in free radical levels.[242] One very recent discovery about resveratrol may have long ranging implications. A group of naturally occurring enzymes in all organisms, called sirtuins, appears to play a significant role in metabolism, aging, and gene expression. Sirtuins act as a deacetylase (they remove acetyl groups) from histones, the molecules that cover genes. In essence, sirtuins silence gene expression, hence the name silent information regulator (Sir 1, Sir 2, Sir 3, etc.). Unchecked gene expression appears to cause aging. By decreasing gene expression, aging is slowed. It is well known that calorie restriction results in longer lifespan in a variety of species. Sirtuins are now thought to mediate the extension of life associated with calorie restriction.[243,244] It appears that resveratrol activates sirtuins. A remarkable study in 2003 demonstrated that resveratrol increased the lifespan of yeast by 70%.[245] Finally, it is to be noted that resveratrol activates proteasomal function. This activation results in increased disposal of abnormal proteins, such as the amyloid-beta peptides found in AD. This has been proven experimentally but awaits clinical confirmation in patients with AD.[246] Based on the discussion above, resveratrol should also prove beneficial in enhancing proteasomal function in PD. The dosage is 200mg/day taken as a single dose. The contraindication would be in individuals hypersensitive to grape products.

Summary

Based on the discussion above, PD patients should benefit from certain dietary changes and the use of supplements and herbs. Each PD patient is different and requires his or her own individual program. In particular, mildly affected patients will not need as intensive a program as more severely affected patients.

The following recommendations are based on the seven categories of factors, discussed above, affecting PD.

Diet: All PD patients should strive to eat organic produce. This has no pesticides, the lowest level of toxic heavy metals, and the highest concentration of minerals and vitamins, including the antioxidant nutrients. To curb constipation and increase L-dopa absorption from the bowel, increase insoluble fiber by eating wheat or rice bran and ground flax seeds. Also, limit breads, crackers, and cereals to those that are made with whole grains. Dosage for ground flax seed is to build up to 1-2 tablespoons daily. The protein redistribution diet is recommended, particularly if there are any off periods when the L-dopa is ineffective. Consultation with a nutritionist may be necessary to achieve the optimal 5:1(by weight) carbohydrate: protein ratio in the diet.

Toxic exposure: Any ongoing toxic exposure should be eliminated. Organic food, as noted above, should be stressed in the diet because of the lesser amounts of toxic metals, herbicides, and pesticides. Some water-soluble fiber, such as psyllium or ground flax seeds, should be added to the diet along with the vitamins and minerals known to aid in liver detoxification. These nutrients, such as calcium, magnesium, zinc, and chromium, can be taken best in a high quality vitamin-mineral supplement. Avoid supplements with iron and copper because of their deleterious roles in PD. The sulfur containing amino acids aid in liver detoxification and can be added to the diet with a protein supplement powder. Garlic and onions are also a nutritious way to increase sulfur in the diet. An herbal extract with milk thistle is recommended for PD patient liver health and if there is a history of increased toxic exposure, schizandra is also indicated. Schizandra probably is best used when there is toxic exposure or some type of acute illness involving fatigue or respiratory involvement. We have not recommended it clinically for long-term use in PD. Milk thistle also reduces xanthine oxidase activity, thus reducing free radical formation. Dosages are 175mg twice/day for milk thistle and 500-1000mg/day for schizandra. If there is a possibility of significant toxic exposure, a heavy metal screening with hair, urine or blood, or after a DMPS challenge should be considered. If positive, a full detoxification program should be considered. A physician specializing in detoxification, or integrated medicine in general, can be very helpful at this point. Practitioners can be found by contacting the American College for the Advancement of Medicine, the American

Holistic Medical Association, or the International Society for Orthomolecular Medicine.

Oxidative stress: The vitamin-mineral supplement recommended above also should have high dosages of vitamins C and E, and beta-carotene for antioxidant protection. Optimal daily dosages have not been established but 1000mg of vitamin C, 200-600 IU of vitamin E, and 25,000 IU of beta-carotene are appropriate. It is important to use the d-alpha tocopherol, or natural, form of vitamin E. Also, it is essential to use a product that contains mixed tocopherols, the class of molecules constituting vitamin E, which may be as important if not more important than alpha-tocopherol for certain functions in the body. Because of the importance of antioxidant protection in PD and the recent discoveries about alpha-synuclein, one should consider using NAC, an antioxidant and precursor of GSH, 500mg twice/day on an empty stomach. NAC also helps with detoxification and reduces nitric oxide production. Sustained release alpha-lipoic acid, 300mg/day, is also recommended for its prominent antioxidant benefits. Finally, melatonin has antioxidant properties and may be particularly valuable in neurodegenerative disorders. Dosage is variable but 1mg at bedtime should be adequate. Milk thistle also may be considered for antioxidant adaptation. Dosage is 175mg twice/day. IV GSH treatment may be considered and obtained from an MD with a holistic or integrated practice.

Dopamine: Early in Parkinsonism, the availability of dopamine is not as urgent as later in the disease. For moderate PD, particularly if on-off effects are present, consider adding NADH, 5mg twice/day, to increase dopamine production. If there is little response to NADH, consider trying nicotinamide, 500mg twice/day, a precursor of NADH. It also acts as a free radical scavenger (antioxidant). If there are side effects from L-dopa, consider adding 5-hydroxytryptophan, 50mg two to three times/day, to raise brain serotonin levels.

Solaray's product, DopaBean, contains 50mg of L-dopa. This supplement has the advantage of the antioxidant properties of the additional constituents in the preparation but lacks carbidopa. Addition of carbidopa may be considered. Dosage depends upon the individual's response to the herb but the equivalent dosage of L-dopa in DopaBean to the individual's current prescribed L-dopa dosage is reasonable.

Excitotoxicity: Magnesium blocks the NMDA receptor, diminishing the injurious effects of glutamate, the excitatory neurotransmitter. Supplementing with magnesium, 200mg twice/day, is indicated. This amount may be in the multivitamin-mineral supplement. Magnesium has the added benefit of alleviating constipation if this is an issue. Increased intake of the amino acid citrulline or use of Huperzine A, both inhibitors of glutamate production, may be considered. Citrulline is found in watermelon and the dosage for Huperzine is 50-200mcg twice/day. To inhibit glutamate production, supplementation of branched chain amino acids L-leucine, L-isoleucine, and L-valine may be possible by using specific protein supplements or by eating brown rice. Taurine, due to its multiple benefits in reducing excitotoxicity is recommended at a dosage of 500mg twice/day on an empty stomach. Avoid using Viagra.

Mitochondria: CoQ10 is an important supplement in PD. It repairs the deficiency in the electron transport chain in the mitochondria. This improves cellular energy, which in turn protects the brain cells from oxidation and other forms of toxicity. In addition, CoQ10 is important for immune and cardiac function and can be helpful in hypertension and diabetes mellitus. Traditional dosages (100-200mg/day) need to be modified considering that the recent University of California, San Diego study revealed 1200mg/day of CoQ10 slowed the progression of the disease and improved motor function. A schedule of 300mg of CoQ10 at breakfast, lunch, dinner, and bedtime is suggested. Ginkgo biloba, 60mg twice/day, appears to protect complex I against injury although it may need to be supplemented under physician supervision as discussed at the end of Section 6.

Alpha-synuclein: As noted above, NAC blocks the clumping together of the abnormally folded alpha-synuclein proteins. NAC, an important naturally occurring antioxidant in the body, has a number of important applications as a supplement in neurology. It increases GSH, the main intracellular antioxidant, protects mitochondria, and appears to protect against the toxic effects of mercury in certain circumstances.[247,248] It is recommended in PD for its various benefits at a dose of 500mg twice/day on an empty stomach. Avoid pesticides as they have been shown to stimulate formation of alpha-synuclein fibrils. This further emphasizes the necessity of eating organic foods.

Inflammation: It is essential for PD patients to use their diet, herbs, and supplements to inhibit the inflammatory process. Taking 500-1000mg/day of EPA plus DHA, omega-3 fatty acids found in fish oil, in liquid or gel capsules is indicated. Nordic Naturals and Carlson Laboratories are safe sources for fish oil, which needs to be free of detectable levels of pesticides and heavy metals. For those individuals on a processed-free, organic diet, GLA may be utilized. It generally comes with linoleic acid with a total dosage of both GLA and linoleic acid of 250-500mg/day. GLA is found in borage oil, black currant seed oil and evening primrose oil.

Herbs to consider for reducing inflammation are baikal skullcap, turmeric, feverfew, ginger, green tea, holy basil, nettle leaf, oregano, and rosemary. Other extracts that may be helpful are bromelain, up to 2400GDU two-four times/day, Nexrutine (250mg/day), the Ayurvedic herb Boswellia, and the extract of the Chinese medicinal herb Atractylodes. Choose these herbs according to personal preference and while taking other medical conditions into account. Turmeric extract, an effective and safe anti-inflammatory and liver tonic, may be taken at 900mg/day. Patients will also benefit from reducing sugar intake.

Ubiquitin-proteasomal system (UPS): Proteasomal function should be enhanced by taking resveratrol. The dosage is 200mg/day taken as a single dose. The contraindication would be in individuals hypersensitive to grape products.

Chapter Two Supplement Chart

Supplement	Dose	Frequency	Instructions
Alpha-lipoic acid	300mg	Day	Sustained release form
Beta-carotene	25000IU	Day	
Bromelain	2400GDU	Two-four times/day	
CoQ10	100-300mg	Up to four times/day	Breakfast, lunch, dinner, bedtime
Fish oil (EPA & DHA)	500mg	One-two times/day	Pesticide and heavy metal free liquid or gel capsules

Supplement	Dose	Frequency	Instructions
Ginkgo biloba	60mg	Twice/day	Use caution with platelet inhibitors or anticuagulants
GLA & Linoleic acid	250-500mg	Day	
Ground flax seed	1-2 tbsp	Day	
Huperzine A	50-200mcg	Twice/day	
Magnesium	200mg	Twice/day	
Melatonin	Up to 1mg	Day	Bedtime
Milk thistle	175mg	Twice/day	
N-acetyl cysteine	500mg	Twice daily	Empty stomach
NADH	5mg	Twice/day	
Nexrutine	250mg	Day	
Nicotinamide	500mg	Twice/day	
Resveratrol	200mg	Day	Not for patients sensitive to grape products
Schizandra	500-1000mg	Day	Acute treatment only
Taurine	500mg	Twice/day	Empty stomach
Turmeric	900mg	Day	
Vitamin C	1000mg	Day	
Vitamin E	200-600IU	Day	D-alpha tocopherol; mixed tocopherols

Chapter Three

Alzheimer's Disease

Alzheimer's disease (AD) is the most common degenerative disease of the brain and causes slowly progressive dementia. The social impact is significant with an overall incidence of almost 5% of people over sixty years of age. The incidence increases with age reaching almost 11% new cases per year in individuals over eighty years of age. The major symptom is a gradual onset of forgetfulness for names, words, and day-to-day events. Ability to use language, arithmetic, and spatial orientation may slowly deteriorate. Judgment and personal hygiene may decline and delusions or hallucinations may occur. Late in the course of the disease, the patient may forget how to use common, everyday tools or utensils and develop mild difficulty with ambulation. Variation in presentation may evade diagnosis early on.

Diagnosis involves brain imaging, either with computed tomography (CT) or magnetic resonance imaging (MRI) scans, blood tests, a brainwave test (electroencephalogram (EEG)), and sometimes neuropsychological testing. It is important to rule out depression since elderly depressed individuals can appear demented. Blood tests help rule out kidney, liver, thyroid, and metabolic disorders. Multiple strokes (infarcts), tumors, vitamin deficiencies, syphilis,

AIDS, and enlarged ventricles with excess cerebrospinal fluid (hydrocephalus) are other potential causes of dementia. There are other neurodegenerative disorders such as Pick's Disease and Lewy Body Disease that cause dementia and need to be considered in the differential diagnosis.

In AD, the brain tends to shrink with loss of brain cells, particularly in a memory related area called the hippocampus. Abnormal fibers known as neurofibrillary tangles are found inside of nerve cells and there are deposits called senile plaques, made of an amorphous protein (amyloid), in the spaces between neurons. Degeneration of other brain cells occurs in a form called granulovacuolar degeneration, again most prevalent in the hippocampus.

The main constituent of amyloid plaques is beta-amyloid, derived from a much larger protein called the amyloid precursor protein (APP). Enzymes or proteases called alpha, beta, and gamma secretases cleave the APP molecule, normally bound to nerve cell membranes, into different length amyloid-beta molecules. An abnormal 42 amino acid length residue tends to deposit into the senile plaques. A gene error in familial AD codes for proteins called presenilins, which may be gamma secretase, the secretase thought to be abnormal in AD. On chromosome 21, familial cases may also have a gene error coding for an abnormal amyloid precursor protein.

The toxicity of amyloid-beta 42 includes the induction of oxidative stress, disturbance of intracellular calcium ion homeostasis,[249] lipid peroxidation, glutamate uptake, and uncoupling of a G protein-linked receptor (membrane signaling transducer proteins).[250] Cholinergic neurons (manufacturing acetylcholine as a neurotransmitter) are affected at very low dosages of beta-amyloid, explaining the particular involvement of the basal forebrain cholinergic system in AD. The activation of proinflammatory microglia, reactive astrocytes and certain cytokines (messenger substances) is associated with beta-amyloid deposition. The induction of oxidative stress includes increases in proinflammatory enzymes such as cyclo-oxygenase-2 and phospholipase (resulting in increased arachidonic acid) suggesting the activation of pro-inflammatory genes.[251]

The neurofibrillary tangles noted above are composed of a normal tau protein that has become hyperphosphorylated (extra phosphate groups). Tau is a cytoskeletal protein which may promote the assemblage of microtubules in nerve cells and may also bind iron and deliver it to nerve cells. There are enzymes, called protein phosphatases, PP-2A and PP-2B, which can convert the hyperphosphorylated tau protein to its normal state. Their activity is decreased in brains of AD patients.[252] Of interest is that aluminum and zinc, both implicated in AD, and arachidonic acid all polymerize the hyperphosphorylated tau into the neurofibrillary tangles.

Another complicating feature of the disease is the affinity of apolipoprotein E, a regulator of lipid metabolism, for beta-amyloid protein. There are several forms (isoforms) of apolipoprotein E produced by different gene alleles on chromosome 19. The presence of one E4 gene allele triples the risk of AD and the presence of two E4 alleles makes the disease highly likely in people surviving into their eighties. The E4 isoform (APOE) also decreases the age of onset and intensifies all the biochemical disturbances in AD including amyloid deposition, tangle formation, neuronal cell death, oxidative stress, and dysfunction of cholinergic signaling.[253] In contrast, other isoforms of apolipoprotein E may be protective.

Other abnormalities exist as well. Neurotransmitters are reduced in AD. These include acetylcholine, noradrenaline, Gamma-aminobutyric acid (GABA), serotonin, and glutamate. In addition, neuropeptide transmitters including substance P, somatostatin, and cholecystokinin are decreased. There is a 30% reduction in glucose metabolism but this is possibly secondary to the loss of neurons rather than a primary problem.

1. Antioxidants and Anti-inflammatory Agents

As noted above, beta-amyloid causes free radical production, which results in oxidative stress to all surrounding molecules, particularly lipids. This oxidative stress is associated with an inflammatory process with activated microglia, cytokines, and other inflammatory markers. There are a number of nutrient approaches to reducing this cascade of events in AD.

N-Acetyl-Cysteine: N-Acetyl-Cysteine (NAC) is derived from the amino acid cysteine in the body. It is a source of sulfhydryl groups and is metabolized into compounds that stimulate glutathione (GSH) synthesis and act as antioxidants and free radical scavengers. Sulfhydryl groups, consisting of sulfur and hydrogen, are essential in much of human metabolism and the function of enzymes, other types of proteins, and ribonucleic acid (RNA). GSH, consisting of cysteine, glutamic acid and glycine, is a critical antioxidant for the brain. NAC is used for treatment of toxicity from acetaminophen, carbon monoxide, heavy metals, and various other exogenous toxicities. It is used as well for a large group of disorders including angina, amyotrophic lateral sclerosis (ALS), Sjogren's syndrome, and alcoholic liver damage.

A study in Switzerland showed that NAC down-regulated gene transcription of amyloid precursor protein (APP) in human neuroblastoma cells.[254] Reducing APP levels could decrease the formation of amyloid plaques. This property, along with its anti-inflammatory action, may explain the positive results obtained, in a subset of cognitive measures, when AD patients were treated with NAC as part of a 2001 study.[255]

NAC can cause some gastrointestinal (GI) side effects. It can reduce carbamazepine drug levels, affect blood test levels of chloride and creatinine, and perhaps rarely raise liver enzymes. In general it is a safe supplement. A starting dose for AD would be 200mg twice/day on an empty stomach. Depending upon the response, working up to 500mg twice/day may be considered.

Turmeric: It is established that chronic use of non-steroidal anti-inflammatories reduces the incidence of AD. They appear to reduce the aggregation of A-beta (amyloid-beta-peptide) fibrils and also to suppress activity of microglia (the brain's inflammatory cells).[256,257] Unfortunately, chronic use of these medications, such as ibuprofen and naproxen, can cause GI damage and liver and renal toxicity. However, many of the benefits of anti-inflammatories may be obtained by using turmeric, which contains antioxidants including the polyphenol curcumin. An experimental study at UCLA showed that curcumin lowered oxidized proteins in the brains of experimental mice used for their tendency to develop AD pathology. Curcumin reduced interleuken-1beta (a pro-inflammatory cytokine), insoluble and soluble beta-amyloid, and plaque burden by 43-50%. Activation of microglia was also reduced.[258] Further support for use of turmeric comes from a 2004 in vitro study that showed a dose-dependent reduction in beta-amyloid fibrils in response to treatment with curcumin.[259]

Turmeric may cause GI side effects long term. If bloating, gas, nausea, or indigestion occur, stop the turmeric. It can be retried at a later date. In theory, turmeric could increase the risk of bleeding, particularly when used with platelet inhibitors such as aspirin. Turmeric dosage is 900mg/day of a standardized extract.

Vitamins E and C: A study at the University of Kentucky showed that Vitamin E reduced protein oxidation, reactive oxygen species formation, and neurotoxicity of the 42 amino acid amyloid-beta-peptide in rat embryonic hippocampal neuronal culture.[260] Low cerebrospinal fluid concentrations of vitamins C and E are observed in AD patients and a 2002 study revealed diminished intakes of antioxidant vitamins, including vitamins E and C, in AD patients.[261] A clinical study in La Jolla with AD patients indicated that vitamin E "may slow functional deterioration leading to nursing home placement in AD patients."[262] These results are supported by a multi-center clinical trial that revealed vitamin E treatment (2000IU/day) significantly slowed disease progression comparable to results obtained with selegiline.[263] A combination of vitamin E with vitamin C may be necessary for optimal results, as noted in a German study that found a decrease in lipoprotein oxidation only when patients took both vitamins.[264] This result is predictable from the known dependence of antioxidants on each other for their sustained efficacy.

Appropriate dosages of vitamins C and E seldom cause side effects. However, vitamin E slightly increases the risk of bleeding, particularly when combined with antiplatelet drugs, such as aspirin, Plavix, or Aggrenox. 200-600IU/day of vitamin E and up to 1gm/day of vitamin C is appropriate in AD. It is important to use d-alpha tocopherol, the natural form of vitamin E. Also, it is essential to use a product that contains mixed tocopherols, the class of molecules constituting vitamin E, which may be as important if not more important than alpha-tocopherol for certain functions in the body. It should be added that the best way to take antioxidants is in combination with each other rather than taking one by itself. A high potency multivitamin generally provides substantial amounts of antioxidants. Vitamins E and C can then be added to increase the daily dose.

Alpha-lipoic acid: Alpha-lipoic acid (ALA) is a very useful antioxidant. It is both water and fat-soluble, enters the nervous system easily, reduces vitamins C and E from their oxidized state (making them reusable), and increases intracellular levels of GSH, a critical intracellular antioxidant. Dosage for ALA is 300mg/day of a sustained release formulation.

Pycnogenol: Pycnogenol, an extract from the bark of the French maritime pine tree, contains important antioxidant flavonoids. Flavonoids are compounds with multiple beneficial effects on health, and are found in plants, fruits, vegetables, and some beverages. A study at Loma Linda University revealed that Pycnogenol suppressed the generation of reactive oxygen species in a rat pheochromocytoma cell line exposed to beta-amyloid. Pycnogenol also suppressed other events that lead up to programmed cell death (apoptosis) that occurs in AD. These events included caspase-3 activation and DNA fragmentation as well as suppressing apoptosis itself.[265] Pycnogenol also protects animal brain cells from the excitotoxicity of high levels of glutamate, a neurotransmitter that plays a role in neurodegenerative disorders.[266]

Because of preliminary evidence that Pycnogenol stimulates the immune system, the one potential theoretical concern with its use is when the individual has an autoimmune disorder. Pycnogenol dosage is 50-100mg three times/day.

Garlic: The same group from Loma Linda University studied aged garlic extract using the same technique as was used with Pycnogenol. The garlic suppressed the same events as Pycnogenol, including the generation of reactive oxygen species, fragmentation of DNA, and apoptosis.[267] Garlic has been used safely for many disorders although it can cause GI side effects. It can enhance the effect of coumadin and in theory, could interact with antiplatelet drugs. It may interact with antidiabetic agents, cyclosporine, AIDS medication, and oral contraceptives. Garlic has potential effects on the hepatic enzyme cytochrome P450 3A4 (CYP450) so an individual should determine if he or she is on a medicine that is metabolized by this enzyme. This enzyme metabolizes approximately half of the pharmaceuticals such as the statin drugs Lipitor and Pravachol and the hormone estradiol. Patients are advised to determine how their medication is metabolized because a potential interaction exists between the metabolism of the medication and garlic. Garlic dosages vary from 600mg three times/day up to 7.2gm/day.

Ginkgo Biloba: Ginkgo biloba is the world's oldest living tree species with a medicinal history dating back to the oldest Chinese material medica (2800 BC). It has a number of beneficial pharmacologic effects. It is an antioxidant, a free-radical scavenger, a vasodilator, and an inhibitor of platelet activating factor. This latter effect decreases platelet aggregation, phagocyte chemotaxis, smooth muscle contraction and excitatory amino acid receptor function. This compound effect of decreasing platelet activating factor results in better cerebral circulation, less inflammation and less excitotoxicity. These are all beneficial effects in AD.

Multiple studies show that Ginkgo biloba protects neurons against beta-amyloid neurotoxicity including reduction of apoptosis.[268,269] It appears to inhibit formation of amyloid fibrils and decrease the activity of caspase 3, a key signaling enzyme in the apoptosis cascade.[270]

Numerous clinical studies show benefit of Ginkgo biloba in AD. This includes the statistically significant results of three recent American studies.[271,272,273] Improvement was seen in cognitive and social spheres with no significant side effects. A recent study in Zurich revealed the effect of Ginkgo biloba was comparable to four cholinesterase inhibitors, the current standard drug therapy for AD.[274] Ginkgo biloba has minimal side effects including effects on blood coagulation. It can magnify the effects of coumadin and platelet inhibitors. Preliminary evidence suggests that it may affect several of the P450 hepatic enzymes. This could lead, in theory, to an effect on the metabolism of a number of pharmaceutical drugs. *The Natural Medicines: Comprehensive Database* discusses this in detail.[18] Ginkgo biloba dosage is 120mg/day, divided into 2-3 separate dosages.

Melatonin: Melatonin is a hormone secreted by the pineal gland, which regulates the body's circadian rhythm, endocrine secretions, and sleep patterns. It is produced from the amino acid L-tryptophan by way of 5-hydroxytryptophan, serotonin and N-acetylserotonin. There is evidence that it has an anticancer effect and is a potent antioxidant. It may be six to ten times more potent than vitamin E as an antioxidant. It neutralizes oxygen-derived free radicals and carbon-centered free radicals. Multiple studies reveal that melatonin significantly reduces the lipid peroxidation secondary to beta-amyloid.[275,276] In cell culture, melatonin also inhibits the secretion of beta-amyloid precursor protein.[277] This information suggests a potential benefit of melatonin in preventing or slowing the progression of AD.

Side effects from melatonin are mild but possibly include sedation. It may increase blood pressure in patients on antihypertensive medications. Some minor drug interactions occur that are listed in the *Natural Medicines Comprehensive Database*.[278] Some interactions are potentially beneficial. Melatonin dosage range is 0.3 to 5mg at bedtime.

2. Homocysteine

Homocysteine is an amino acid produced by the body and elevated levels are associated with heart attacks, stroke, and hardening and narrowing of the arteries. Folic acid and vitamins B12 and B6 support the natural breakdown of homocysteine and consequently the lowering of blood homocysteine levels. Conflicting information exists regarding the role of elevated plasma homocysteine in AD. A 1998 *Archives of Neurology* study found significantly higher homocysteine levels and reduced vitamin B12 and folate levels in AD patients.[279] Disease progression was higher in the patients with higher homocysteine level at the beginning of the study. A 1999 study at University of California, Davis reported significantly higher homocysteine levels in 164 AD patients than in a control group of elderly individuals with no cognitive impairment.[280] A 2002 report from Princeton University notes that homocysteine globally decreases brain methylation, an important metabolic process for structural components and neurotransmitters. Methylation is essential for protein phosphatase 2A(PP2A) heterodimer formation, which dephosphorylates tau protein. The researchers postulated that elevated homocysteine reduces PP2A methylation leading to tau hyperphosphorylation, which is central to AD pathology.[281] Finally, a 2002 study at Oxford University revealed homocysteine to be an independent risk factor for white matter hypodensity (leukoaraiosis) on CT scans.[282] This latter study is significant for AD because lack of cerebral blood flow, or ischemia, is commonly associated with AD. Reduced density (hypodensity) on a CT scan is suggestive of impaired circulation to the hypodense area. A 2002 study in *Neurology* found significant elevations of homocysteine in AD patients only when there was associated vascular disease.[283] This study and another done in 2002 suggest that increased homocysteine levels are a risk factor for vascular disease in patients with AD.[284] This is consistent with the fact that patients with AD are at known risk for vascular disease. Homocysteine may play a role in AD, either in AD pathology or in associated vascular disease. Homocysteine levels are easily reduced with folate, and vitamins B6 and B12. A good multi-vitamin or a B-complex, with dosages of 1mg for folate, up to 100mg of B6, and 1000mcg for B12 is indicated. Use methylcobalamine for B12.

3. Neuronal Cellular Structure and Function

Phosphatidylserine: Phosphatidylserine (PS) is the most abundant phospholipid in the human brain and is important in maintenance of the cellular internal environment, signal transduction, secretary vessel release, cell-to-cell communication and regulation of cell growth. Although manufactured in the body, most PS is dietary in origin. PS increases acetylcholine, norepinephrine, serotonin, and dopamine in animal models and patients with AD. In animals PS appears to reduce age-related neuronal dendrite loss and atrophy of cholinergic neurons.[285]

Several studies show significant improvement in cognition associated with PS treatment in both normal elderly and AD patients.[286,287,288,289] It is well tolerated with possible side effects of GI upset or insomnia. There are no significant drug interactions. PS dosage is 100mg three times/day.

Acetyl-L-carnitine: Acetyl-L-carnitine (ALC) occurs naturally in the body in the inner membrane of mitochondria, the powerhouses of cells. It serves as a mitochondrial precursor to acetyl coenzyme A (acetyl CoA), which contributes acetyl moieties for acetylcholine. It has several other cholinergic enhancing properties including promotion of acetylcholine release from cells and increasing choline acetyltransferase, an enzyme involved in acetylcholine formation. It is also a carrier of long-chain fatty acids from the cytoplasm into the mitochondria thereby enhancing mitochondrial energy production. It enhances synaptic transmission, increases hippocampal binding of nerve growth factor and reduces age-related losses of hippocampal glucocorticoid receptors. It appears to increase cerebral blood flow in individuals with cerebrovascular disease.[290] A recent study also demonstrated that ALC inhibited the neurotoxic effects of beta-amyloid, suggesting another mechanism for its benefit in AD.[291]

Several studies show benefit of ALC in AD patients.[292,293,294,295] It may cause GI side effects and agitation. It has no drug interactions. Dosage in AD varies from 500-2000mg/day divided into two doses.

4. Neurotransmitters

As noted above, neurotransmitters decline in AD, probably secondary to neuronal injury and loss. Current pharmaceutical treatment of AD involves inhibition of cholinesterase, the enzyme that hydrolyzes acetylcholine, the most salient neurotransmitter for memory. Cholinergic neurons are particularly affected in AD. In addition to the pharmaceutical agents such as Exelon (rivastigmine) and Aricept (donepezil hydrochloride), supplements may be helpful as well.

Acetyl-L-carnitine: please see the discussion above regarding cholinergic enhancement by ALC

Huperzine A: Huperzine A is an alkaloid isolated from the Chinese club moss, Huperzia serrata. It crosses the blood-brain barrier and is a reversible inhibitor of acetylcholinesterase (AChE), the enzyme that breaks down acetylcholine. It may be more specific for AChE and have a longer duration of action than the pharmaceutical agents noted above. In animals, Huperzine A was sixty-four times more potent than Cognex (tacrine) and may be more bioavailable and more effective at crossing the blood-brain barrier.[296] Other favorable properties include inhibition of the neurotoxicity of beta-amyloid[297] and reduction of glutamate-induced apoptosis by blocking N-methyl-D-aspartate (NMDA) ion channels.[298] Results from a 2004 study showed Huperzine A lasted longer and increased cortical acetylcholine levels eight and two times more than donepezil and rivastigmine, respectively.[299] Huperzine A, donepezil, tacrine, rivastigmine, and physostigmine were compared in a 2002 report that showed each to be significant inhibitors of different molecular forms (G1 and G4) of AChE in different rat-brain regions (cortex, hippocampus, and striatum).[300] Other studies have shown significant AChE inhibition with hybrids of Huperzine A and tacrine (huprines).[301,302]

Several studies confirm the efficacy of Huperzine A in human subjects without significant side effects.[303,304,305] It may cause nausea, sweating, blurred vision and other cholinergic side effects although it is thought to have fewer side effects than the comparable pharmaceuticals. It might interfere with anticholinergic drugs and have an additive effect to cholinergic agents such as the drugs for myasthenia gravis. Dosage for AD varies from 50-200mcg twice/day.

5. Essential Fatty Acids

Docosahexaenoic acid (DHA), a long-chain polyunsaturated Omega-3 essential fatty acid, has important central nervous system (CNS) functions including playing a key role in development of retinal, neuronal, and synaptic membranes and support of learning, memory, and cognition. Long-chain fatty acids make up one-third of all lipids in the brain's gray matter, the region containing neuronal cell bodies. A comparison of AD patients and individuals with no cognitive impairment showed the AD patients had significantly lower DHA levels. This 2003 study also showed lower levels of DHA were associated with more severe dementia.[306] A 2002 study in Japan demonstrated that DHA had multiple beneficial effects in a rat model of AD. DHA markedly diminished the loss of avoidance learning ability in rats administered beta-amyloid into the cerebral ventricles. There was a decrease in apoptotic products, an increase in reduced GSH levels and reduced lipid peroxides and reactive oxygen species.[307]

DHA has a high concentration in fish oil. A teaspoon/day, or gel capsules, with dosages of EPA plus DHA from 500-1000mg/day is suggested. When using fish oil, choose a product that states it has been assayed and found free of heavy metals and organic toxins such as pesticides and herbicides. If GI upset occurs, take the product with food and confirm its freshness by checking the expiration date on the bottle.

6. Aluminum

The role of aluminum in AD remains controversial despite the known elevation of aluminum in AD brains, the epidemiological association of increased AD incidence in areas with elevated aluminum in drinking water, and the biochemical mechanisms linking aluminum with AD pathology. By 2001, nine out of thirteen epidemiological studies demonstrated a positive correlation between municipal water aluminum levels and AD.[308] Aluminum can present as elemental aluminum or in multiple organic forms.

Injection of aluminum into animals produces neuropathological and neurochemical changes in the CNS similar to the changes seen in AD.[309] Aluminum produces these changes in multiple ways. It promotes formation of insoluble beta-amyloid and hyperphosphorylated tau. It facilitates iron-induced oxidative injury and disrupts calcium regulation. It may activate reactive oxygen species and initiate inflammatory processes mediated by inflammatory cytokines.[310,311] Increased aluminum in the diet of mice increased beta-amyloid levels and accelerated plaque formation, which was reversed by vitamin E.[312]

Although not definitive, the evidence strongly suggests a role of aluminum in AD and the need to avoid excess consumption and exposure. Many antiperspirants and some cookware contain aluminum and should be avoided. In addition to the consumption of pure water, avoiding antacids and certain analgesics is paramount. Some antacids contain many thousand times the amount of aluminum compared with drinking water. David Perlmutter, in his book *BrainRecovery.com* presents an extensive list of antacids and analgesics containing aluminum.[313] The reader is recommended to his book for this information.

7. Glycation End Products

Glycation is the abnormal reaction of sugars with amino groups of proteins and occurs as part of the aging process. Glycated proteins form abnormal cross-linkages with multiple secondary effects. They activate intracellular information pathways leading to increased production of inflammatory signaling molecules, called cytokines, and free radical production with increased oxidative stress. This ultimately leads to damage of multiple cellular components.[314] Cross-linking may occur in the formation of beta-amyloid and hyperphosphorylated tau. Advanced glycation end products (AGE) also activate glial cells to produce free radicals such as the superoxide radical and nitric oxide as well as the neurotoxic cytokine, tumor necrosis factor-alpha (TNF-α).[315] Carnosine is found in multiple tissues and is a naturally occurring di-peptide (beta-alanine and L-histidine) that inhibits AGE formation. Carnosine levels decline with age. In addition to reducing AGE, carnosine has antioxidant effects, binds heavy metals, and may reduce copper and zinc induced neurotoxicity. No drug interactions are known to occur and there are no reported side effects. Carnosine dosage is 500mg twice/day.

8. Electromagnetic Fields

Multiple studies support the relationship between exposure to electromagnetic fields and the occurrence of AD;[316,317,318] however, two studies show no significant relationship.[319,320] It is postulated that electromagnetic fields may influence calcium homeostasis and activate immune system cells such as CNS microglial cells. In a 2003 study, researchers concluded electromagnetic fields from cell phones alter brain function due to energy absorption. Cell phones placed near rabbits' heads, in a manner that simulated the electromagnetic field exposure received by a human during normal cell phone use, caused significant changes in brain electrical activity in nine of the ten animals studied.[321] The effect was not seen when the phone was moved away from the brain, at the level of the chest. It is important to avoid excessive electromagnetic field exposure including cell phones, transmission lines, and occupational equipment, particularly in individuals at risk for AD.

9. Vitamin D

Patients with AD have an increased risk for falls and hip fractures. A study in Japan in 1998 found reduced bone mineral density and vitamin D and ionized calcium levels in AD patients. Other evidence suggested that the patients were sunlight deprived and suffered from malnutrition, leading to the vitamin D and calcium deficiencies.[322] This study underscores the importance of sun exposure and vitamin D and calcium supplementation. Although the dosage for vitamin D generally varies with age, 1000IU is a reasonable dosage. Dosage for calcium is 500-1500mg/day. Higher dosages should be used if a bone density scan indicates osteopenia or osteoporosis.

10. The Proteasome

A more complete discussion on the proteasome and its role in neurodegenerative disorders may be found in the chapter on PD. In summary, the proteasome is a barrel-shaped organelle in every cell that is responsible for the digestion of protein. Homeostasis, or maintenance of balance, is just as important in the life of every cell as it is maintaining a checkbook or keeping our house clean. Proteins are constantly being manufactured in each cell for enzymatic, structural and other purposes. Cellular housekeeping requires the disposal of used protein. This is accomplished by the attachment of a protein called ubiquitin to the protein, which results in the protein being digested in the barrel shaped multi-protein structure called the proteasome. Research demonstrates diminished function of the proteasome in AD. Multiple studies suggest that the proteins accumulating in AD, namely amyloid and paired helical filaments, inhibit the proteasome, which may, in turn, become increasingly incapable of digesting proteins related to the accumulation of these insoluble protein aggregates.[323,324,325] Resveratrol, a polyphenol found in grapes and red wine is known to stimulate proteasomal function. This is discussed at greater length in the PD chapter. In addition, a recent study demonstrated that resveratrol markedly lowered both the amount of secreted amyloid-beta and intracellular amyloid-beta, the protein found in the amyloid plaques of AD. Various experiments appear to prove that the reduction was related to increased activity of the proteasome.[326] Resveratrol is a very safe supplement used at a dosage of 200mg/day.

Summary

The selection of herbs and nutrients will vary depending upon a number of factors. For healthy individuals concerned about a genetic risk of AD, the selection would differ from an individual known to have two APOE 4 alleles through genetic testing. Finally, the choices may involve an individual with known AD, either early or late in its course. Under any circumstances, individuals may benefit from eating organic foods and supplementing with vitamins, minerals, antioxidants, and essential fatty acids because it is well established, with voluminous data from the U.S. Department of Agriculture, that our food is moderately to severely depleted in nutrients. This relates to the severe loss of topsoil, lack of crop rotation, the use of pesticides and herbicides, and early harvesting from the plants. It is also well established that the essential fatty acids in our food supply is significantly altered. Since the nervous system is primarily fat, the quality of our essential fatty acid intake is very important for the health of the nervous system, as well as our body as a whole.

Diet: All AD patients should strive to eat organic produce. This has no pesticides, the lowest level of toxic heavy metals, and the highest concentration of minerals and vitamins, including the antioxidant nutrients.

A high quality multivitamin-mineral supplement: A high quality multivitamin is usually an encapsulated powder with chelated minerals and the absence of additives. The encapsulated powder is preferable also because it is difficult for the gastrointestinal system to digest and absorb the nutrients in a one-a-day vitamin tablet. The dosing for encapsulated nutrients is generally 2-3 capsules twice/day. The optimal amounts of nutrients cannot easily be compressed into a single capsule or tablet that is absorbable. Inorganic forms of minerals are often used in tablets and additives often are present to aid in manufacturing, shelf life, and appearance. Single tablet vitamins are best avoided unless a high quality company specially manufactures them for this purpose. B vitamins are important to reduce homocysteine levels and the antioxidant vitamins E and C should be present in adequate amounts. The multi-vitamin may need to be supplemented with a B complex for a total dosage of 1mg of folate, up to 100mg of B6 and 1000mcg of B12. If necessary, supplement vitamin E for a daily total of 200-600IU and vitamin C to 1gm/day. Vitamin E may increase the risk of bleeding, especially if combined with drugs that effect bleeding. It is important to use d-alpha tocopherol, the natural form of vitamin E. Also, it is essential to use a product that contains mixed tocopherols, the class of molecules constituting vitamin E, which may be as important, if not more important, than alpha-tocopherol for certain functions in the body. Calcium, 500-1500mg/day and vitamin D, 1000IU/day, as well as regular sun exposure are helpful to increase bone mineral density.

Essential fatty acids: One of the more important essential fatty acids for the brain is DHA. Fish oils are high in DHA. Unfortunately, fish contain significant levels of mercury, prompting an FDA advisory against consumption of tuna, king mackerel, swordfish, tilefish, and shark by pregnant women, newborns and young children. Taking 500-1000mg/day of DHA plus EPA in liquid or gel capsules is indicated. Nordic Naturals and Carlson Laboratories are safe sources for fish oil supplements, which need to be free of detectable levels of pesticides and heavy metals. Essential fatty acids from vegetable sources, such as flaxseed oil, a tablespoon/day are also beneficial, although only a very small amount is metabolized in the body to DHA, one of the more important essential fatty acids for the brain.

Antioxidants and anti-inflammatory agents: Aging stresses the body's antioxidant system. The following antioxidants and anti-inflammatory agents are recommended to help prevent, manage symptoms of, and slow the progression of AD: NAC on an empty stomach, starting at 200mg twice/day and depending upon the response, working up to 500mg twice/day. NAC may cause GI side effects, reduce carbamazepine drug levels, effect blood test levels of chloride and creatinine, and rarely raise liver enzymes.

Dosage for standardized turmeric extract is 900mg/day. This may cause GI side effects if used long-term. If this happens, discontinue use and resume at a later date. Turmeric may increase the risk of bleeding, particularly when used with platelet inhibitors such as aspirin. Vitamins E and C are important antioxidants and are discussed above in the multivitamin section. ALA dosage is 300mg/day of a sustained release formula and Pycnogenol dosage is 50-100mg three times/day. Individuals with autoimmune disorders should not use Pycnogenol. Garlic, 600mg three times/day to 7.2gms/day, is safe for many disorders but can cause GI side effects, enhance the effect of coumadin, and interact with antiplatelet drugs, antidiabetic agents, cyclosporine, AIDS medication, and oral contraceptives. It also has potential effects on medications, such as antidepressants and antiseizure medications that rely on CYP450 for metabolism. *Natural Medicines: Comprehensive Database* is a resource for drug interaction information.[327] Recommended dosage for Ginkgo biloba is 120mg in two or three divided dosages/day. Gingko biloba can affect blood coagulation and magnify the effects of coumadin and platelet inhibitors, and interact with drugs that rely on P450 hepatic enzymes for metabolism. Melatonin, which can be sedating and may increase blood pressure in patients on antihypertensive medications, can be taken at bedtime with a dosage of 0.3-5mg/day. Individual preferences and other health factors should help you with the selection of a particular antioxidant.

Cell structure and function and neurotransmitters: To support the neuronal environment and enhance neurotransmitter function, take PS, 100mg three times/day, acetyl-L-carnitine, 500-2000mg/day in two divided dosages, and Huperzine A, 50-200mcg twice/day. All three of these treatments may cause GI upset, and Huperzine A may cause sweating, blurred vision, and other cholinergic side effects, although fewer than that caused by pharmaceuticals. Huperzine A may have an additive effect on cholinergic agents and may interfere with anticholinergic drugs. To support proteasome function, resveratrol 200mg/day is recommended.

Aluminum, glycation end products, electromagnetic fields, monosodium glutamate (MSG), and aspartame: Avoid ingestion of and exposure to aluminum, which can be found in some antacids, drinking water, cookware, and antiperspirants. Take carnosine, 500mg twice/day, to reduce advanced glycation end products, bind heavy metals, and as an antioxidant. Avoid exposure to electromagnetic fields from cell phones, transmission lines, and occupational equipment. MSG and aspartame should be avoided.[328,329]

Chapter Three Supplement Chart

Supplement	Dose	Frequency	Instructions
Acetyl-l-carnitine	500-2000mg	Day	Two divided dosages
Alpha lipoic acid (ALA)	300mg	Day	Sustained release
Calcium	500-1500mg	Day	
Carnosine	500mg	Twice/day	
Fish oil (EPA & DHA)	500mg	One-two times/day	Pesticide and heavy metal-free liquid or gel capsules
Folate	1mg	Once/day	
Garlic	Up to 4gm	Day	See summary for cautions

Supplement	Dose	Frequency	Instructions
Ginkgo biloba	120mg	Day	In two-three divided dosages
Huperzine A	50-200mcg	Twice/day	See summary for cautions
Melatonin	0.3-5mg	Day	Bedtime
Multivitamin-mineral	Follow instructions on label	Follow instructions on label	Encapsulated powder
N-acetyl cysteine (NAC)	200-500mg	Twice/day	Empty stomach
Phosphatidyl-serine	100mg	Three times/day	
Pyncogenol	50-100mg	Three times/day	Not for individuals with autoimmune disorders
Resveratrol	200mg	Day	
Turmeric	900mg	Day	
Vitamin B6	Up to 100mg	Once/day	
Vitamin B12	1000mcg	Once/day	Use methylcobala-mine
Vitamin C	1gm	Day	
Vitamin D	1000IU	Once/day	
Vitamin E	200-600IU	Day	Use D-alpha tocopherol with mixed tocopherols

Chapter Four

Atherosclerosis and Stroke

Atherosclerosis, the degenerative hardening of blood vessels that occurs with aging, is thought to be the leading cause of death and disability in developed countries. It can affect the coronary blood vessels, leading to a heart attack; the brain's circulation, causing stroke; and the blood vessels of the limbs, causing claudication and even gangrene. Stroke is the loss of brain function associated with blockage of blood to a specific brain region. Atherosclerosis tends to occur at blood vessel branching points such as the bifurcation of the common carotid artery into the internal and external carotid arteries in the neck. It generally develops over many years with a long silent period prior to the clinical manifestations such as heart attack and stroke.

The development of atherosclerosis is complex and affected by risk factors of elevated lipids such as cholesterol and triglyceride, high blood pressure, diabetes, smoking, elevated homocysteine levels, and a positive family history. For simplicity, the development of atherosclerosis resulting in stroke is divided in this chapter into a sequence of processes, which in fact are totally interdependent on each other. Separating the process into component parts clarifies how various supplements and medications can affect specific stages of atherosclerosis.

Endothelial dysfunction: Dysfunction of the endothelium, the cells lining the inner channel of arteries, may be the earliest abnormality in the development of atherosclerosis. The endothelium has many secretory, metabolic, and immunologic functions. It produces information molecules, such as nitric oxide, that regulate blood flow. It also affects platelet aggregation and adhesion to the vessel wall, and the balance between the clotting (coagulation) and unclotting (anticoagulation or fibrinolysis) of blood. The endothelium secretes substances that both promote and inhibit the growth of vascular smooth muscle cells. Dysfunction of the endothelium may be defined as an imbalance between the chemical mediators for vessel relaxation and contraction, blood coagulation and anticoagulation, and growth promoting and inhibiting factors. The risk factors of hypertension, diabetes, smoking, and elevated lipids, such as cholesterol, result in early dysfunction of the endothelium, an initiating event in atherosclerosis.[330]

A number of recent studies suggest that damaged endothelial cells may have diminished formation of nitric oxide (NO), a small gaseous particle that has many functions in the body. It is formed by the amino acid L-arginine and nitric oxide synthase, an enzyme that is diminished in atherosclerosis.[331] In addition to being a vasodilator, NO inhibits oxidation of the low-density lipoprotein (LDL) form of cholesterol. Vitamin C has been shown, in animal studies, to have a protective effect on endothelial function by increasing nitric oxide synthase activity, resulting in increased NO levels.[332] A number of recent studies demonstrate that statins, a group of drugs that inhibit an enzyme, 3-Hydroxy-3-methylglutaryl coenzyme A

(HMG-CoA) reductase, and are used primarily to lower cholesterol and LDL, increase the concentration of nitric oxide synthase. This results in increased cerebral blood flow and reduced infarct (damaged tissue) size in experimental animals.[333,334,335] The statins may have other antiatherosclerotic effects, which are discussed below. Red yeast rice, which contains a natural statin-like compound and has antioxidant properties, will be discussed as well.

There are other molecules that play a role in later stages of atherosclerosis when blood coagulation complicates the atherosclerotic plaque (the fatty lesion of atherosclerosis) on the inner wall of arteries. Some of the factors, including von Willebrand factor, fibrinogen, tissue plasminogen activator, plasminogen activator inhibitor, and adhesion molecules, are derived from endothelial cells. Plasminogen is a precursor of plasmin, a molecule that promotes the breakdown, or lysis, of clots. Plasminogen is strongly bound to fibrin, the molecule that polymerizes blood constituents to form a clot. Fibrinogen is a well-established risk factor in stroke. One study demonstrated an almost six-times greater risk in individuals with fibrinogen levels over 407mg/dl. There was also a significantly increased risk of plaque rupture in patients with elevated fibrinogen values.[336] A 2004 British study also demonstrated a linear increase in stroke risk with fibrinogen levels in patients post transient ischemic attack (TIA) or minor ischemic stroke.[337] Nattokinase (NK), a protein derived from fermented soybeans, acts as a fibrinolytic (breaking down fibrin) enzyme and has been studied in animals. These studies have suggested it has potential for use in atherosclerosis and stroke when there is evidence for hypercoagulation including elevated levels of fibrinogen, the molecular precursor of fibrin.[338] NK has been shown, in animal studies, to significantly reduce clot size and to have four times the ability of plasmin to break down fibrin.[339,340]

Although there is no direct evidence at this time for its use in atherosclerosis and stroke, it may be of benefit to patients with hypercoagulation, which has been associated with aging and disorders such as chronic fatigue syndrome and fibromyalgia.[341] In those cases, NK may be considered at a dose of 2000 fibrin units/day. It should be used with close physician supervision.

Chronic endothelial injury and lipids: Following the early endothelial dysfunction, there may be loss of endothelial cells. This allows platelets to stick to the extracellular matrix underneath the endothelial cells. This leads to formation of chemotactic factors, messenger molecules that attract inflammatory cells. It also causes platelets to release growth factors that promote smooth muscle cell replication in the vessel wall, narrowing the inside of the vessel. In tandem, oxidized LDL, toxic to endothelial cells, increases endothelial injury. LDL is called the bad cholesterol primarily because of its injurious effects on vessel walls. It is prone to oxidation by free radicals, a pervasive process in the body. The LDL particles accumulate in the inner lining of the vessel (the intima), and contribute to the recruitment of inflammatory cells and smooth muscle growth. Eventually, a mature atherosclerotic plaque forms with a lipid core containing both intracellular and extracellular lipid, areas of calcification, and a fibrous cap composed of collagen.

Alpha-lipoic acid (ALA) and N-acetyl cysteine (NAC) can be used to reduce several atherosclerosis risk factors, such as oxidative stress, inflammation, production of adhesion molecules, and elevated homocysteine levels. ALA, an important antioxidant, prevents the bonding of sugar to proteins (protein glycosylation), a process contributing to aging and to complications in diabetes mellitus. These bonded end products are called advanced glycation end products (AGEs) and they stimulate the expression of adhesion molecules. In order for inflammatory molecules to adhere to the vessel wall, they must attach to an adhesion molecule such as vascular cell adhesion molecule-1 (VCAM-1). By reducing AGEs, ALA reduces VCAM-1 expression, thereby reducing the inflammatory response in atherosclerosis.[342] ALA has numerous other properties suggesting its use in this setting. It is both water and fat soluble and can recycle the vitamin E contained in LDL, thus boosting antioxidant activity.[343] Another study showed that ALA augmented glutathione (GSH) and vitamin C levels that had been diminished by AGEs. GSH is an essential intracellular antioxidant. The researchers also found GSH and vitamin C reduction activated a transcription factor, nuclear factor-kappa B (NF-kappa B), which plays a role in the development of atherosclerosis. Transcription factors are information molecules that control the activity of various genes. This study showed ALA also reduced NF-kappa B activation.[344] Dosage for ALA is 300mg/day in a sustained release form.

A study in Haifa, Israel, showed that pomegranate wine, red wine and NAC inhibited NF-kappa B activation in vascular endothelial cells.[345] This may explain, in part, the benefit of red wine in reducing cardiovascular disease. NAC, a derivative of the amino acid L-cysteine, appears to reduce both homocysteine[346] and lipoprotein(a),[347] two risk factors for atherosclerosis. NAC has a number of other therapeutic benefits such as increasing production of GSH, dissolving mucous in respiratory ailments, protecting the liver from acetaminophen toxicity, and helping with mercury detoxification. Finally, by inhibiting the enzyme that breaks down the matrix of an atherosclerotic plaque, NAC appears to help prevent plaque destabilization, an event that can precede stroke.[348] These studies suggest the use of NAC, 500mg twice/day on an empty stomach, in atherosclerosis and stroke.

Reduction of cholesterol and oxidized LDL: The progression of atherosclerosis can be slowed by lowering cholesterol levels, particularly the LDL form, as well as by decreasing the oxidation of LDL. Raising high-density lipoprotein (HDL) levels is also of benefit because HDL transports cholesterol from the periphery back to the liver and directly protects the blood vessel wall. HDL also interferes with a number of processes in the atherosclerotic plaque, including the binding of LDL and inflammatory white blood cells and the oxidation of LDL. The following discussion addresses several nutrients that have been shown to reduce oxidation of LDL, lower cholesterol and LDL, and raise HDL.

- **Coenzyme Q10 (CoQ10):** CoQ10, also known as ubiquinone, is a vital intermediate in a cellular process called the electron transport chain. This last step in the conversion of our food into energy, or adenosine triphosphate (ATP), takes place in the mitochondria, small organelles inside each cell. Low levels of CoQ10 are also found in the LDL of plasma, the fluid part of blood. It is thought that CoQ10 is an important antioxidant defense for LDL particles.[349] An Australian study demonstrated that oral CoQ10 supplementation alone or in combination with vitamin E made plasma lipids more resistant to peroxidation induced by peroxyl radicals. Of interest is that vitamin E alone, a known antioxidant, did not offer this benefit. In the mice used in the study, vitamin E, CoQ10, or the combination reduced aortic atherosclerosis, with the combination of vitamin E and CoQ10 showing reduction over the longest distance of the aorta, the main artery leaving the heart. Only the combination reduced the percent of oxidized lipid in the aortic tissue itself.[350] These results are supported by the findings of three other studies;[351,352,353] however, a 2002 German study found only ambivalent benefits for CoQ10 in hyperlipemic rabbits and a negative effect for vitamin E.[354] It is difficult to conclude with certainty the application of these results in humans. It is known that antioxidants act as components of a system in the body, requiring each other for a sustained effect. It is not advisable to take a single antioxidant, such as vitamin E, by itself, without other antioxidants such as vitamin C, CoQ10, and ALA. It is advisable to take vitamins E and C along with ALA. Adding CoQ10 provides additional benefits. More human studies, although difficult to fund, are strongly encouraged by the animal data.

It should be added that the HMG-CoA reductase inhibitors or statins, such as Lipitor or Pravachol, reduce serum levels of CoQ10.[355,356] Because statins reduce the synthesis of mevalonate, a substrate needed for CoQ10 synthesis, production of CoQ10 may drop by as much as 25-40% with statin treatment.[357] Results from a 2003 study of three different statins and forty-two patients indicated a dose dependent reduction in plasma CoQ10 with statin treatment.[358] For this reason, the authors of that study recommended administration of CoQ10 to minimize the adverse effects of statins. CoQ10 is also advised for its other benefits including the enhancement of cellular energy production. This property in turn explains its value in congestive heart failure, neurodegenerative disorders, and the possible prevention of cancer. Dosing for CoQ10 is 100mg once-twice/day

- **Vitamin E:** It has been established that in aging adults, higher plasma vitamin E levels are significantly related to a reduction in risk for cardiovascular events. Researchers from Italy separated their participant data into four groups, from lowest to highest, based on vitamin E plasma levels. Individuals in the group with the highest vitamin E levels had one-sixth the cardiovascular risk compared with individuals in the group with the lowest vitamin E levels.[359]

  Vitamin E is a group of compounds called tocopherols and tocotrienols. Tocotrienols are antioxidants derived from plants, such as palm fruit, and have even more antioxidant power than tocopherols. Tocopherols are oily, yellow liquids found in the lipids of plants in leaves, seeds and other parts. Vitamin E is known to be transported in the LDL particles and is recycled by vitamin C and ALA. A recent study demonstrated that three tocopherols (alpha, gamma and delta) were comparable in increasing active nitric oxide synthase, the formative enzyme of nitric oxide discussed above. Protection against lipid peroxidation was similar as was inhibition of platelet aggregation. The combination of the three tocopherols had a synergistic effect. Li and his co-authors suggest that clinical trials with commercial preparations of only alpha-tocopherol may explain the inconsistent results seen in the vitamin E literature.[360] A 2002 study in Sweden confirmed that mixed tocopherols had a stronger inhibitory effect on lipid peroxidation than alpha-tocopherol alone. This may explain why the consumption of mixed tocopherols in food protects against atherosclerotic cardiovascular disease whereas alpha-tocopherol supplementation alone does not have a significant effect.[361] Further evidence suggesting the need for combining antioxidants and taking mixed tocopherols comes form a Harvard University study of 43,738 health professionals that did not reveal a protective effect of vitamin E on the incidence of stroke.[362] Similarly, a study at University of Southern California in 2002 demonstrated that alpha-tocopherol lowered oxidized LDL but did not alter the course of atherosclerosis as measured by ultrasonography.[363] These studies again reiterate that supplementation with a single antioxidant may be ineffective, or worse, deleterious, when it becomes oxidized. Similar to CoQ10, vitamin E taken with other antioxidants is suggested in atherosclerosis for its general health benefits.

Another benefit of vitamin E is the reduction of C-reactive protein levels. C-reactive protein lowers levels of nitric oxide synthase, an enzyme that is diminished in atherosclerosis.[364] Statin drugs, the current accepted group of cholesterol lowering agents, also lower C-reactive protein levels. Atherosclerosis, as noted above, has a strong inflammatory component and C-reactive protein plays a significant part in inflammation. A process called the acute phase response plays an important role in inflammation. It may be initiated by an information molecule called interleukin-6, which has been shown to decrease with vitamin E supplementation.[365] Interleukin-6 causes a cascade of events with the initial secretion of C-reactive protein, fibrinogen, and serum amyloid A. These molecules incite an inflammatory response. These results further suggest the use of vitamin E for atherosclerosis. A mixed tocopherol (alpha, gamma, and delta) preparation is strongly recommended based on the studies noted above. It is important to use d-alpha-tocopherol, the natural form of vitamin E. The dosage for vitamin E is 200-600IU/day.

- **Vitamin C:** Vitamin C levels are known to be inversely related to total cholesterol and triglyceride levels and proportionate to HDL levels, particularly unoxidized HDL. A recent study from Slovakia demonstrated that homocysteine, a risk factor for atherosclerosis and stroke, has been shown to have levels inversely correlated with plasma vitamin C.[366] Experimentally, vitamin C restores depleted GSH and decreases DNA and protein damage in vascular smooth muscle cells.[367] Finally, a six-year study with 136IU of vitamin E and 250mg of vitamin C twice/day revealed a significant reduction in carotid artery atherosclerosis demonstrated by ultrasound.[368] Vitamin C is recommended at a dosage of 500mg twice/day in combination with other antioxidants as mentioned above.

- **Policosanol:** Policosanol is a mixture of cane sugar alcohols, the largest percent of which is octacosanol, a 28-carbon long-chain alcohol. Policosanol appears to reduce the cellular expression of HMG-CoA reductase, an essential enzyme in cholesterol production. The statin drugs such as Lipitor work by inhibiting this enzyme versus the down-regulation of its presence by Policosanol.[369] Policosanol also inhibits platelet aggregation, another potential benefit in prevention of atherosclerosis.[370]

Multiple animal studies reveal significant effects on reducing atherosclerotic lesions in animals. A 1995 study in Cuba found that Policosanol significantly reduced the occurrence of atherosclerotic lesions in rats.[371] A subsequent study in rabbits, fed a cholesterol rich diet, found that the control group developed marked hypercholesterolemia and lesions of atherosclerosis with thickening of the intima, the inner layer of arteries affected early-on in atherosclerosis. In most rabbits treated with Policosanol, atherosclerotic lesions were not present and intimal thickening was significantly less than in controls.[372]

A series of human studies suggest the efficacy and safety of Policosanol in improving lipid profiles; however, these studies have been of only Cuban populations and with Cuban-produced Policosanol, which is not available in the U.S. A 1999 study compared Policosanol with pravastatin (Pravachol), a common statin drug used to lower cholesterol levels. Policosanol significantly lowered LDL 19% compared with 16% with pravastatin. Total cholesterol decreased 14% with Policosanol compared with 12% with pravastatin. Only Policosanol significantly raised HDL levels and it was by 18%. No side effects were reported on Policosanol.[373] Another study by the same group compared Policosanol (10mg/day) and lovastatin (Mevacor)(20mg/day). Policosanol lowered LDL 20% compared with 17% with lovastatin, and Policosanol raised HDL by 8%. Lovastatin raised muscle and liver enzymes in some patients. No side effects were reported in the Policosanol group.[374] Results from 2002 placebo-controlled study showed 5mg/day of Policosanol lowered LDL 21%, total cholesterol 15%, and triglyceride 12% and increased HDL 13%. Vascular and all-cause serious adverse events were significantly lower in the Policosanol than the control group. Policosanol was also found to significantly decrease blood pressure. No significant side effects were noted.[375] While these results are promising, further research is needed to determine if similar results will be obtained in other populations and with non-Cuban Policosanol. Dosage for Policosanol may be considered at 5-10mg/day.

- **Red yeast rice (Monascus purpureus):** Red yeast rice is prepared according to an ancient method of fermenting the fungal strain Monascus purpureus on moist, sterile rice. The important metabolites belong to a group of chemicals called the monacolin family of polyketides. Fatty acids and trace elements are also present.[376] A 2002 study in Hong Kong found that Cholestin, a proprietary brand of red yeast rice, inhibited cholesterol levels in a system of hepatic (liver) cells. It directly inhibited 69-78% of HMG-CoA reductase activity, the enzyme inhibited by all statin drugs.[377]

  Multiple clinical studies have shown the efficacy of red yeast rice in reducing cholesterol, LDL cholesterol, and triglycerides while raising HDL cholesterol. A 1999 double-blind, placebo-controlled study at University of California, Los Angeles found total cholesterol decreased from an average of 254mg/dl to 208mg/dl. The LDL cholesterol dropped from an average of 175 to 135. Triglyceride levels dropped significantly as well. HDL did not change significantly. No serious adverse effects were noted.[378] Three other clinical studies confirmed significant lowering of cholesterol, LDL cholesterol, and triglycerides with two studies showing significant elevations in HDL cholesterol. Combining the four studies, the cholesterol decrease varied from approximately 16 to 26%, LDL cholesterol from 21% to 30% and triglyceride from 11% to 34%. Two studies showed HDL increases of approximately 20% and 15%. No significant toxicity was seen in multiple studies.[379,380,381] Long-term users should consider checking liver function tests. Standard red yeast rice dosage is 600mg once or twice/day. Because of variation in standardization and other issues, the authors recommend Choleast by Thorne. Standard dosage is 2 capsules twice/day. Lipid profiles should be monitored.

- **Niacin:** The vitamin niacin (nicotinic acid and niacinamide) is essential for a number of metabolic reactions in the body. In addition, it has been the subject of many studies in hyperlipidemia, excessive fats (cholesterol and triglycerides) in the blood. It is unique in that it favorably affects all lipid abnormalities by reduction of total cholesterol, triglyceride, and LDL cholesterol, while raising HDL cholesterol levels. It also reduces lipoprotein(a), a known risk factor for atherosclerosis.[382] It has been shown to promote regression of coronary artery disease and decrease coronary events, stroke, and total mortality.[383] A comparative study of niacin and lovastatin, a common lipid-lowering drug, was conducted in a group health foundation in Minnesota.

Although LDL decreased 26% with lovastatin and 18% with niacin, HDL increased only 2% with lovastatin but increased 16% with niacin. Triglyceride decreased 8% with lovastatin and 18% with niacin.[384] Niacin has several interesting antiatherogenic properties. There are various proteins, called apolipoproteins, that carry lipids in the HDL and LDL particles. The HDL particles that have the A-I apolipoprotein are more protective against atherosclerosis than those with the AII apolipoprotein. A study at the Long Beach, California Veterans Administration hospital demonstrated that niacin, unlike gemfibrozil, a cholesterol lowering agent, selectively increased the fraction of HDL particles containing the A-I apolipoprotein.[385] Niacin also shifts the LDL profile towards the large buoyant particles and away from the more atherogenic small dense particles.[386,387]

Niacin is available in simple vitamin form, sustained-release form, and an extended-release form, called inositol hexaniacinate. Flushing is a common side effect of the simple vitamin form and hepatotoxicity has been seen with the sustained-release form. The extended release form (inositol hexaniacinate) has a reduced incidence of flushing and no significant liver side effects. Inositol hexaniacinate consists of six niacin molecules attached radially to the sugar inositol. It is thought to be comparable to niacin in its benefits on the lipid profile, although fewer studies are available than for niacin itself. The dosage of niacin is one 1-4 grams/day.

- **Pantethine:** Pantethine, or vitamin B5 (pantothenic acid), is an essential component of Coenzyme A (CoA), involved in the transport of fats to and from cells. Pantethine is known to lower elevated lipids including triglyceride. It may inhibit HMG-CoA, similar to the statins, reducing cholesterol levels. Its metabolite, cystamine, inhibits hepatic acetyl-CoA carboxylase. Acetyl-CoA carboxylase is a hepatic enzyme that adds CO_2 (carbon dioxide) to molecules to create longer chain fatty acids, particularly triglycerides. By inhibiting this enzyme, cystamine appears to lower the synthesis of triglycerides.[388] Dosing for pantethine is 600-1200mg/day in divided doses, under medical supervision.

- **Garlic:** By enhancing antioxidant potential in the blood and decreasing lipid peroxidation, garlic has been shown to suppress atherosclerosis in animal studies.[389,390,391] Aged garlic has been shown to lower both total and LDL cholesterol. An Australian study of rabbits, fed a cholesterol-enriched diet, revealed that Kyolic, an aged garlic extract, reduced the surface area of aortic atherosclerosis by 64%. It also appeared to inhibit proliferation of vascular smooth muscle cells.[392] A study at Loma Linda University showed that S-allyl cysteine, a component of garlic, inhibited LDL oxidation, hydrogen peroxide radical formation, and NF-kappa B activation.[393] As discussed above, NF-kappa B is an intracellular information molecule that is involved in the formation of atherosclerosis. The Loma Linda findings suggest that garlic inhibits multiple mechanisms related to atherosclerosis. Garlic contains an amino acid called alliin. When crushed, the alliin in the garlic clove comes in contact with an enzyme allinase, converting the alliin to allicin. Multiple studies demonstrate the lipid lowering effect of allicin.[394,395,396] It is important to use a garlic supplement that supplies a high allicin potential. Garlic dosage for elevated cholesterol is 400-600mg once-twice/day. This dosage should supply at least 10mg of alliin, with an allicin potential of at least 4000mcg.

- **Gugulipid:** Gugulipid is the standardized extract of the mukul myrrh tree, native to India. The active agents in gugulipids affect bile acid molecules that regulate cholesterol levels.[397] A 1994 study with 50mg twice/day of gugulipid reduced total cholesterol by approximately 12%, LDL cholesterol 13% and triglyceride by 12%. Lipid peroxides, a measure of oxidative stress declined 33%. A few patients experienced headache, mild nausea, eructation, and hiccup.[398] A multi-center, 205 patient clinical trial of gugulipid showed significant reduction in total cholesterol, triglycerides, and LDL, and an increase in HDL in 70-80% of the patients.[399] Patients taking propanolol or diltiazem for blood pressure should not take gugulipid because it reduces the bioavailability of these two drugs.[400] Gugulipid should be standardized to an important constituent, guggulsterones. Total guggulsterone percentage is usually 10%. An effective dose is 50-100mg of total guggulsterones daily.

- **Dietary Fiber:** Dietary fiber is the indigestible components of fruits and vegetables. It consists of polysaccharides, long chains of sugar molecules linked together. The molecular structure determines whether the fiber is cellulose, hemicellulose, pectin, lignin, gums, or mucilage. By increasing the bulk of fecal material, intestinal transport is quickened, and toxins are removed more quickly from the body.

Dietary fiber reduces several risk factors related to stroke as well as the incidence of stroke itself. It is well established that it reduces elevated cholesterol levels.[401,402,403] Although mild, the effect is significant and includes a reduction in the bad cholesterol, LDL. In addition, dietary fiber appears to reduce circulating levels of C-reactive protein, a known risk factor for heart attack and stroke.[404,405] A 2000 study in Boston revealed that increased intake of whole grains was associated with a lower risk of ischemic stroke in women.[406] Whole grains contain the bran as well as the endosperm and germ of the grain. The bran is rich in fiber, B vitamins and trace minerals. It is the only part of the grain that contains fiber. A study at Harvard University in 1999 revealed that diets high in fiber, potassium and magnesium reduced the risk of stroke.[407] In addition, dietary fiber lowers the risk of coronary heart disease, an indirect risk for stroke.[408]

In addition to changes in diet, various supplements are available containing dietary fiber. One good example is Dr. Richard Schulze's Intestinal Formula #2. It contains several sources of fiber, including flax seed, apple pectin and psyllium seed. It also contains some Bentonite clay and activated willow charcoal. Bentonite clay is known to draw toxins, including heavy metals, from the gut, to be excreted from the body. Activated charcoal also has a reputation for absorbing cholesterol as well as environmental toxins and its use has been the standard of practice in emergency rooms in the treatment of intake of poisons and overdose of various pharmaceuticals.

Renin-angiotensin system: In 1898, researchers found they could raise blood pressure using a kidney tissue extract. The substance, named renin, acts as an enzyme that converts a plasma protein, angiotensinogen, secreted by the liver, to angiotensin I. Angiotensin I is converted by an enzyme, called angiotensin converting enzyme (ACE), into angiotensin II, which is the pressure elevating form of angiotensin.

Angiotensin II constricts blood vessels, increases sympathetic nervous system tone, increases sodium reabsorption from the kidney, causes release of another potentially hypertensive substance, aldosterone, from the adrenal cortex, and alters renal blood flow. Recent studies demonstrate additional effects including the promotion of inflammation and cell proliferation through signal cascades which contribute to atherosclerosis.[409] These latter effects explain the observed benefit of two new classes of drugs, ACE inhibitors and angiotensin receptor blockers (ARB), in atherosclerosis.

Natural approaches are available for reduction of angiotensin. A study last year demonstrated that vitamin D (1,25-dihydroxyvitamin D(3)) significantly inhibited the genetic expression of renin production, which would lead to lower angiotensin levels.[410] This explains the well known relationship between reduced sunlight exposure and high blood pressure and elevated renin levels.[411] Vitamin D can be safely used up to 4000IU/day although it is unlikely that dosages this high would be necessary for the renin-angiotensin effect. A daily dosage of 400IU of vitamin D is generally recommended. If your serum 25-hydroxy vitamin D level is low, taking up to 1000IU/day is suggested.

Several studies have demonstrated the ACE inhibiting properties of plants. A study in Denmark evaluated thirty-one plant species traditionally used for blood pressure control and found that seven inhibited ACE activity by over 50%.[412] A 2001 study in France examining three plant species demonstrated that flavonoids, including proanthocyanidins, inhibited ACE.[413] In particular, they studied hawthorn (Crataegus oxycantha), a classic heart tonic herb. Hawthorn has other benefits in this setting including antioxidant activity, increasing coronary blood flow, strengthening myocardial contraction, and improving lipid profiles.[414] Dosage depends upon the concentration of the extract. If standardized to 1.8% vitexin-4-rhamoside, the dose is 100-250mg three times/day. If standardized to 18% procyanidolic oligomers, dose is 250-500mg/day.

Platelets: Drugs that inhibit platelets are commonly used in atherosclerotic disease and its complications, such as myocardial infarction (heart attack) and stroke. The standard drugs include aspirin, Ticlid (ticlopidine), Plavix (clopidogrel), and Persantine (dipyridamole). The first three reduce the incidence of myocardial infarction (MI) and stroke although ticlopidine and clopidogrel are more effective than aspirin. Aspirin inhibits an enzyme, cyclooxygenase, which in turn reduces the formation of thromboxane A2 (TXA2). TXA2 induces platelet aggregation and vasoconstriction. Ticlopidine and clopidogrel inhibit platelet aggregation by reducing the secretion of adenosine diphosphate (ADP), a molecule required for platelet aggregation. Dipyridamole inhibits platelet uptake of a molecule called adenosine. Through a cascade of events, this inhibition results in reduced aggregation of platelets. Newer therapies involve the combination of platelet inhibitors such as aspirin and Aggrenox (dipyridamole).

The role of platelets in atherosclerosis involves multiple information molecules and a complex interaction with endothelial cells, the inner lining of blood vessels. Platelets and endothelial cells manufacture adhesion molecules, responsible for binding of white blood cells to the endothelium (an important step in atherosclerosis). In addition, platelets appear to manufacture amyloid precursor protein (APP), known for its role in AD. Macrophages, essential inflammatory molecules, consume platelets, and convert APP into beta-amyloid protein, with a resultant inflammatory cascade accelerating atherosclerosis.[415] This parallels the process in AD, reinforcing evidence for inflammation's significant role in numerous disease processes. Platelets activate smooth muscle cell expression of thrombospondin, which appears to provoke smooth muscle cells in vascular walls to proliferate.[416] Smooth muscle cell proliferation is an essential step in atherosclerosis. Finally, platelets secrete a factor called platelet factor 4 (PF4), which binds to oxidized LDL and increases oxidized LDL binding to vascular cells and macrophages. It also appears to block the binding and degradation of non-oxidized LDL, thereby leading to increased oxidized LDL levels.[417]

Ginkgo biloba, the Maidenhair tree, is the oldest living tree species, dating back 200 million years. Extracts of the leaves have a number of properties that suggest their utility in atherosclerosis and stroke. It is a potent inhibitor of a phospholipid, platelet activating factor (PAF), which promotes platelet aggregation and has a broad range of effects in a variety of tissues.[418] PAF appears to act on a specific cell receptor, initiating intracellular signaling processes which ultimately effect gene transcription. It contributes to inflammation and, in a 2002 report, induced death of the main structural cell in the central nervous system (CNS), the glial cell.[419] PAF is found in atherosclerotic plaques and appears to play an important role in atherosclerosis.[420] Gingko extracts may inhibit other atherosclerotic molecular processes noted above. This includes inhibiting the toxic effects of beta-amyloid[421] and preventing the adhesion of inflammatory cells to endothelial cells that line the lumen of blood vessels.[422] Gingko biloba appears to reduce the proliferation of vascular smooth muscle cells[423] and inhibits the activation of NF-kappa B by hydrogen peroxide,[424] both processes essential to atherosclerosis.

Experimental and clinical work on Ginkgo biloba extracts confirms its utility in cerebrovascular disease. Animal studies have shown significant reduction in infarct (stroke) size and increased cerebral blood flow associated with daily administration of Ginkgo biloba.[425] Caspase-3, an intracellular messenger involved in apoptosis (programmed cell death), was less abundant in mice treated with Ginkgo biloba.[426] A Japanese study in stroke-prone, spontaneously hypertensive rats revealed that Ginkgo biloba administration suppressed age related hypertension and reduced thrombotic potential. Another beneficial effect of Ginkgo biloba was that endothelial nitric oxide synthase messenger RNA was significantly higher, which suggests increased vascular nitric oxide production. Measurement of a marker of oxidation was also reduced, suggesting a significant antioxidant effect of Ginkgo biloba.[427] A 2002 study also noted Ginkgo biloba's ability to preserve mitochondrial ATP synthesis and stabilize brain cell membranes exposed to hypoxia (oxygen deprivation). It also increases certain subunits of the electron transport chain (COX III subunit of cytochrome c oxidase and the ND1 subunit of NADH ehydrogenase), the mitochondrial mechanism for energy production.[428]

As of 1992, there were 40 human clinical studies of Ginkgo biloba's effects on cerebrovascular disease. All trials reported positive results although a meta-analysis suggested that only eight studies were well performed.[429] Another meta-analysis in 1994 of 11 placebo-controlled, randomized, double-blind studies found six well-performed studies confirming the efficacy of Ginkgo biloba in cerebrovascular insufficiency.[430] One study in acute stroke patients given Ginkgo biloba starting more than forty-eight hours after the stroke did not show any significant difference compared with a control group. Garg and his co-authors recommend a study in acute stroke starting the Ginkgo biloba within six hours of the stroke.[431] In summary, chronic administration of Ginkgo biloba appears to have a significant protective effect in cerebrovascular disease. Dosage is usually 60mg twice/day. Due to the additive effect of Ginkgo biloba with other platelet inhibitors such as aspirin, Plavix, or Ticlid, and its potential interaction with coumadin, physician supervision is recommended.

Cerebral blood flow, oxygenation and neuroprotection: Vinpocetine, synthesized from the alkaloid vincamine from Vinca minor, may have the broadest application of all supplements in atherosclerosis and stroke. Available since 1978, it has been widely used in Japan, Hungary, Germany, Poland, and Russia.[432] It has multiple actions favorable in the treatment of atherosclerosis and stroke and is taken up preferentially by the CNS.

Vinpocetine appears to protect nerve cells at risk due to inadequate blood supply, after head injury, or in neurodegenerative disorders by blocking sodium channels. One study found it as potent as phenytoin (Dilantin), the widely used anticonvulsant, in blocking sodium channels.[433] Sodium channels are the conduit for entrance of sodium into cells and have been the target for cardiac antiarrhythmic, local anesthetic and anticonvulsant drugs. With significant energy expenditure, every cell membrane has a potential maintained by pumping sodium ions out of the cell. Blocking sodium channels frees up more ATP for other tasks, including protection of the nerve cell in the threatening circumstances noted above.[434] Sodium channel blockade is considered an important neuroprotective property.

Several recent studies demonstrate that vinpocetine increases cerebral blood flow in patients following stroke. A 2002 study in Hungary with near infrared spectroscopy and transcranial Doppler found increased cerebral blood flow and tissue oxygenation with intravenous vinpocetine.[435] A Russian study in 2001 found a significant reduction in stroke morbidity with the acute use of intravenous vinpocetine.[436] Vinpocetine has also been shown to increase uptake and metabolism of glucose in the peri-stroke and healthy brain tissue.[437]

It has been known for years that vinpocetine inhibits a specific type of phosphodiesterase that is dependent on calcium. Phosphodiesterases are intracellular enzymes that metabolize intracellular signaling molecules called cyclic nucleotides. One type, cyclic guanosine monophosphate (cGMP), relaxes vascular smooth muscle. Viagra, the drug for impotency, works by increasing cGMP by inhibiting its specific phosphodiesterase. Vinpocetine increases cGMP by the same mechanism, resulting in vascular dilation and increased blood flow.[438,439] This property of vinpocetine may explain, in part, the benefits in stroke noted above.

A number of studies demonstrate reduced calcification in atherosclerotic tissues in animals fed cholesterol rich diets plus vinpocetine. Using various experimental methods, decreased calcium as well as phosphorus and aluminum were detected in the CNS, kidney, and liver in the experimental animals versus the control animals.[440,441,442] These studies suggest that vinpocetine may inhibit the development of atherosclerosis. Human studies are required to confirm this.

Vinpocetine is recommended at a dosage of 10mg three times/day and is best taken with food.

Homocysteine: Elevated levels of homocysteine are a known risk factor for atherosclerosis. One reason is that it up-regulates collagen (connective tissue) and the accumulation of arterial smooth muscle cells.[443] It also causes endothelial cell dysfunction with impaired regulation of vascular tone, increased recruitment and adhesion of inflammatory molecules to the endothelium, and loss of endothelial cell antithrombotic function (anticoagulation activity).[444] It also induces hyperactivity of platelets, probably via the generation of reactive oxygen species. This may contribute to a thrombogenic state (increased clot formation).[445] These mechanisms help explain the known association of elevated homocysteine levels with carotid artery atherosclerosis[446] and stroke.[447] It is of note that patients on antiepileptic medications[448] and Sinemet (levodopa)[449] may have elevated homocysteine levels, and coffee intake raises levels as well.[450]

Folic acid and vitamins B6 and B12 are involved in the metabolism of homocysteine. Supplementation with these vitamins lowers homocysteine levels[451] and a study is currently underway at Wake Forest University School of Medicine to determine whether supplementation with these vitamins will help prevent recurrent stroke in individuals having suffered a single stroke.[452] The study quoted above utilized 600mcg of folic acid, 800mcg of vitamin B12 and 2mg of vitamin B6. For individuals with known elevation of homocysteine, a B vitamin supplement should be considered.

Exercise: It is important for the reader to note that other lifestyle measures may significantly reduce the risk of stroke. Obesity itself is a risk factor for stroke.[453,454] This may be related to the production of an inflammatory cytokine THF-alpha in fat tissue. This in turn is associated with elevated levels of other inflammatory mediators including C-reactive protein. In addition to weight reduction, exercise has multiple benefits for stroke prevention. It may reduce fibrinogen[455] and C-reactive protein levels.[456] During exercise, muscle produces an anti-inflammatory cytokine, IL-6, which stimulates the production of other anti-inflammatory cytokines, inhibits the production of an inflammatory molecule (tumor necrosis factor alpha or TNF-α), and enhances lipid turnover.[457] Finally, multiple studies have demonstrated a significant reduction in stroke occurrence with physical activity.[458,459,460]

Additional considerations: There are other nutrients to be considered in the overall management of atherosclerosis, its risk factors, and stroke. A recent study showed that flaxseed meal in the diet significantly lowered cholesterol and triglyceride in rats. Soy protein was also beneficial but not to the same degree as flaxseed meal.[461] A 2002 human study at Tufts University showed a modest reduction of cholesterol levels with soy protein.[462] Flaxseed meal and soy protein can be obtained in foods and a recommended daily quantity would be approximately 4-6gm/day, or build up to 1-2 tablespoons/day, of ground flaxseed and 25gm/day of soy protein.

It also has been established that higher consumption of omega-3 fatty acids lowers the risk of coronary heart disease in men and women.[463] A German study demonstrated angiographic regression of coronary disease with omega-3 fatty acid ingestion. These authors also showed omega-3 fatty acids reduced levels of two inflammatory mediators (platelet-derived growth factor and monocyte chemoattractant protein-1) that are involved in atherosclerosis.[464] A 2002 study from England demonstrated that fish oil, taken prior to endarterectomy, affected the nature of the carotid artery plaques. In patients taking fish oil, the fibrous cap of the plaque was thicker and there was less inflammation in the plaque. It is known that atherosclerotic plaques incorporate omega-3 fatty acids. This study demonstrated that increased availability of omega-3 fatty acids resulted in more stable plaques, less likely to rupture and cause an ischemic stroke downstream.[465] Omega-3 fatty acids are found in fish oil, which can be taken as gel capsules at a dosage of 700mg of EPA plus DHA (e.g., 420mg EPA plus 280mg DHA) twice/day. Higher dosages may help reduce triglyceride levels. It is important to use a source for fish oil that is tested to be free of pesticides and heavy metals.

Low levels of two minerals, magnesium and potassium, correlate with increased atherosclerosis, and low intakes of calcium and potassium are associated with hypertension. Low levels of magnesium increase LDL and oxidized LDL concentrations and affect endothelial function.[466] An epidemiological study at Harvard showed that diets rich in potassium, magnesium, and cereal fiber reduced stroke risk, particularly in hypertensive men.[467] A Norwegian study last year showed that reduced potassium levels correlate with increased stroke risk. It was noted that potassium reduces oxidative stress and proliferation of smooth muscle cells, two important elements in the development of atherosclerosis.[468] A reasonable dosage for magnesium is 500mg/day. Calcium requirements depend upon your gender, age and menopausal status. A reasonable pre-menopausal calcium dosage is 1000mg/day. Modest supplementation of potassium in a multivitamin is sufficient.

Padma 28 is a traditional Tibetan herbal formula based on another longevity formula in Tibetan medicine. The formula was transmitted in 1850 from Tibetan monasteries to the Tsar's court of Russia and ultimately to eastern and western Europe, Israel, and the United States. It has been manufactured by Padma Inc., Switzerland with the same formula since 1969. It consists of 20 herbal ingredients combined in a specific order with strict weight ratios. Padma contains multiple phytochemical constituents including polyphenols, flavonoids, saponins, glycosides, glycyrrhizin (found in licorice), terpenoids, and alkaloids. The variety of components account for the system-interactive nature of the formula, which results in a variety of medicinal benefits. This includes antioxidative and anti-inflammatory actions.[469] As discussed in the chapter on multiple sclerosis, Padma 28 has immune-modulatory properties. Another property, which appears to mitigate atherosclerosis, is Padma 28's fibrinolytic action.[470] Padma 28's multiple pharmacological properties help explain its beneficial effects in a variety of disorders including peripheral atherosclerotic disease,[471] angina pectoris (coronary artery disease),[472] chronic hepatitis B,[473] juvenile chronic arthritis,[474] recurrent respiratory infections[475] and multiple sclerosis.[476]

Although a review of Medline does not reveal any controlled studies of Padma in cerebrovascular disease, its known mechanisms of action and its benefit in peripheral and coronary arterial disease recommends its use in atherosclerosis and stroke. In addition to the reduction of the inflammatory, oxidative, and thrombotic processes discussed above, recent studies suggest a particular reduction in lipid oxidation[477] as well as a reduction of multiple pro-inflammatory cytokines.[478] As this chapter describes, the atherosclerotic process is complex, occurring in phases with multiple biochemical mechanisms. The complex properties of Padma, antithetical to the abnormalities in atherosclerosis, as well as the minimal side effect profile, recommend its use in stroke patients with atherosclerosis. Dosage is 2 tablets twice/day.

Summary

The use of nutrients and herbs in atherosclerosis and stroke begins with a thorough medical assessment of risk factors such as abnormal lipids, high blood pressure, diabetes, smoking, and family history, along with other laboratory tests for levels of homocysteine, C-reactive protein, and lipoprotein(a). Assessments of the brain, large vessels, and heart may be important as well. In special circumstances blood tests for a hypercoagulable state may be necessary.

The following appear essential, based on the preceding information, independent of the stage or character of the atherosclerosis and its complications:

A high quality multivitamin-mineral supplement: This will provide the magnesium, potassium, calcium, pantethine, folate, and vitamins B6, B12, C, and E discussed above. A high quality supplement is generally an encapsulated powder without additives, and contains optimal levels of vitamins and organically chelated minerals. Vitamin E should be supplemented at a dosage of 200-600 IU/day. It is important to use d-alpha-tocopherol, the natural form of vitamin E. Also, it is essential to use a product that contains mixed tocopherols, the class of molecules constituting vitamin E, which may be as important if not more important than alpha-tocopherol for certain functions in the body. Vitamin D, which lowers renin production, should be added if not in the multivitamin. 1000 IU/day of vitamin D is reasonable and safe. Vitamin C may need to be supplemented, depending on the content in the multivitamin, for a total dosage of 1000mg/day.

Omega-3 fatty acids: This can be obtained from fish oil. Fish oil, whether by the teaspoon or capsule must be free of heavy metals and pesticides. The product should be independently assayed for these contaminants and state so on the label. Fish oil dosage is 500mg one-two times/day of EPA plus DHA.

Antioxidants: Even in the absence of frank disease, ALA 300mg of a sustained release form is recommended. The need for antioxidant protection in aging is pervasive. In addition, as noted above, ALA interferes specifically with various mechanisms of atherogenesis. CoQ10, 100mg once or twice/day, is advised for its antioxidant, energy producing, and cardiac benefits. In addition, NAC, 500mg two times/day on and empty stomach is suggested.

Hawthorn: Because of its multiple beneficial properties, including ACE inhibition, 250-500mg/day of hawthorn, standardized to 18% procyanidolic oligomers, is recommended. If standardized to 1.8% vitexin-4-rhamoside, the hawthorn dose is 100-250mg three times/day.

Dietary fiber: Include fiber rich foods in the diet, such as vegetables, whole grains, and ground flax seed. Dosage for ground flax seed is to build up to 1-2 tablespoons/day, which increases water-soluble and insoluble fiber levels. Supplements such as Dr. Richard Schulze's Intestinal Formula #2 also may be considered.

In the presence of lipid abnormalities:

Policosanol: Due to limited research, policosanol's efficacy remains to be proven, however it may be considered at 5-10mg/day.

Niacin: Due to its selective effect on LDL and HDL subfractions, niacin should be added. This can be taken as inositol hexaniacinate (the extended-release form) working up as high as 4gm/day. If doses of 2gm or higher are used, liver enzymes should be checked every two-three months.

Red yeast rice: As one of the most effective nutrients for lowering cholesterol, red yeast rice at 600mg once or twice/day is recommended. Similar to the statin drugs, occasional liver function tests should be performed. Lipid profile should be monitored under the care of your practitioner.

Garlic, gugulipid, flaxseed, and soy protein: These can be variably added to the diet. Garlic dosage for elevated cholesterol should provide at least 10mg/day of alliin. Dosage for gugulipid is 50-100mg daily and it should be standardized to 10% total guggulsterone. Policasonal is occasionally combined with gugulipid in the same supplement. Patients taking propanolol or diltiazem for blood pressure should not take gugulipid because it reduces the bioavailability of these two drugs. Flaxseed and soy protein may be taken. The general dosage of ground flaxseed is 4-6gm/day or build up to 1-2 tablespoons/day. Soy protein dosage is approximately 25gm/day.

In the presence of cerebrovascular disease, including stroke:

Ginkgo biloba: There are multiple beneficial properties associated with Ginkgo biloba. Dosage is 120mg/day, in two to three doses, of a standardized product. If bleeding is of concern, the dosage can be lowered to 60mg/day. Due to potential interaction with platelet inhibitors and coumadin,

Ginkgo biloba use should be monitored by your health care practitioner.

Vinpocetine: To increase cerebral blood flow and protect nerve cells, vinpocetine is recommended at a dosage of 10mg three times/day and is best taken with food.

Padma 28: A dosage of 2 tablets twice/day of Padma 28 is recommended for its multiple properties associated with mitigating various factors associated with atherosclerosis.

In the presence of associated chemical risk factors:

Elevated homocysteine levels: Folate 400-600mcg/day, vitamin B6 up to 100mg/day, and vitamin B12 1mg/day. Consider NAC 500mg twice/day on an empty stomach.

Elevated C-reactive protein: Vitamin E (d-alpha-tocopherol plus mixed tocopherols) 200-600 IU/day.

Elevated lipoprotein(a): NAC 500mg twice/day on an empty stomach.

Elevated fibrinogen levels: Nattokinase (NK) may be of benefit at a dosage of 2000 fibrin units per day, under close medical supervision.

Chapter Four Supplement Chart

Supplement	Dose	Frequency	Instructions
Acetyl-l-carnitine	500-2000mg	Day	Two divided dosages
Alpha lipoic acid (ALA)	300mg	Day	Sustained release form

Supplement	Dose	Frequency	Instructions
Calcium	500-1500mg	Day	
Carnosine	500mg	Twice/day	
CoQ10	100mg	Once-twice/day	
Fiber			Follow instructions on label
Fish oil (DHA & EPA)	500mg	Once-Twice/day	Pesticide and heavy metal free liquid or gel capsules
Flax seed, ground	1-2tbsp	Day	
Folate	400-600mcg	Day	
Garlic	400-600mg	Once-Twice/day	Should supply at least 10mg of aliin and allicin potential of 4000mcg
Ginkgo biloba	120mg	Day	In two-three dosages with physician supervision

Supplement	Dose	Frequency	Instructions
Gugulipid	50-100mg	Day	Standardized to 10% total guggulster-one. Do not take with propanolol or diltiazem.
Huperzine A	50-200mcg	Twice/day	
Hawthorn	See summary		
Multivitamin-mineral	Follow instructions on label	Follow instructions on label	Encapsulated powder
N-acetyl cysteine (NAC)	500mg	Twice/day	Empty stomach
Nattokinase	2000 fibrin units	Day	Use only with medical supervision
Niacin	Up to 4gm	Day	Divided into two-three doses; may use inositol hexaniacin-ate, check liver enzymes
Padma 28	2tablets	Twice/day	
Pantethine (B5)	600-1200mg	Day	Divided doses, under medical supervision

Supplement	Dose	Frequency	Instructions
Phosphatidyl-serine	100mg	Three times/day	
Policosanol	5-10mg	Day	
Red yeast rice	600mg	Once-twice/day	Have practitioner monitor lipid profile
Resveratrol	200mg	Day	
Vinpocetine	10mg	Three times/day	Best taken with food
Vitamin B6	Up to 100mg	Day	
Vitamin B12	1000mcg	Day	Use methylcobal-amine
Vitamin C	500mg	Twice/day	
Vitamin D	1000IU	Day	
Vitamin E	200-600IU	Day	Use d-alpha-tocopherol with mixed tocopherols

Chapter Five

Migraine Headaches

Migraine is one of those ills when the body has to bear patiently what the soul cannot.

Dr. Macdonald Critchley,
British neurologist and sufferer of migraine

Migraine generally is an episodic headache which can be disabling. The word migraine is a French version of the Latin word *hemicrania*, meaning half of the skull. This refers to the tendency for migraine to affect one half of the head during an attack. It is estimated that twenty-eight million Americans suffer from migraine with 18.2% of females and 6.5% of males having at least one migraine attack per year. 53% of migraineurs, individuals suffering from migraine, report severe disability or the need for bed rest during an attack. The headache occurs unilaterally 60-70% of the time and the pain is described as throbbing or pulsing with a tendency to become a continuous ache. The headache may be preceded or accompanied by an aura. The aura may be blurred or missing areas in the visual field (scotomas) or positive symptoms, most commonly an arc-like scotoma with a shimmering or glittering zig-zag border. Perception of lights, sparks, or colors may occur. In addition there generally is an increased sensitivity to light (photophobia), sound (phonophobia), and smell (osmophobia). The individual may experience lethargy, mood changes, increased urination (polyuria), soreness and stiffness of neck muscles, anorexia (loss of appetite), and constipation or diarrhea. Tenderness of the scalp as well as firmness and tenderness of scalp vessels are common. More specific neurologic symptoms may occur and the headache may last from four to seventy-two hours.

The understanding and treatment of migraine may date back to the Neolithic period, 7000 years ago, and the use of trephination, creating holes in the skull. In 1200 BCE, Egyptian documents discussed headache and in 400 BCE, Hippocrates described the visual aura that might precede a migraine headache. Multiple ancient and medieval authors addressed the treatment of migraine. Theories variably attributed the cause to a gastrointestinal disorder including colonic toxins, the influence of febrile thoughts, a cerebral allergy, and eyestrain. Over time, modern theories of migraine emerged, divided into vascular and neurogenic etiologies. Based on the clinical observation of vascular and neurologic symptoms, it seemed apparent that the migraine attack involved an episodic disorder of vascular and neurologic systems. One particularly important discovery was made accidentally by Aristides Leao, a graduate student at Harvard in the 1940s. Intending to study epilepsy in an experimental rabbit model, he found that stimulation of the cortex of the rabbit's brain produced a spreading wave of electrical suppression rather than the seizure discharge he expected. This wave propagated at about 3mm/minute. Coincidentally, Karl Lashley, one of the founders of experimental psychology, described his own migraine auras. Applying his own seminal research to himself, he proposed that the slow migration of the scintillating scotoma across his visual field correlated with a propagating neural disturbance in the occipital region of his brain. In addition, the orientation and shape of the fortification pattern, a name applied to the arc of scintillations, suggested an organizing principle of the cortex. Lashley's observation correlated well with Leao's cortical spreading depression (CSD) as well as anticipating the layout of neurons in the visual cortex called iso-orientation domains.

The vascular theory of headaches was advanced by Harold Wolff, a neurologist at Cornell University Medical College in New York City. In the 1930s, Dr. Wolff even performed a craniotomy on a patient during an acute migraine attack. He observed initial vasoconstriction of cerebral vessels followed by vasodilation of extra cranial and intracranial vessels as well as a sterile inflammation of affected vessels. He postulated four phases of migraine: initial vasoconstriction followed by extracranial vasodilation; sterile inflammation; and finally, secondary muscle contraction. He also postulated the presence of vasoactive substances mediating various phases of the migraine attack. Although further experimental studies have found his theory an oversimplified view of migranous events, his seminal work formed a framework for further understanding of the migraine syndrome.

Studies have connected more parts of the migraine syndrome although one unified theory still eludes medical research. Two papers are particularly important. Michael Moskowitz, a professor at Harvard Medical School, reported in 1984 that nervous connections exist between trigeminal ganglia and cerebral blood vessels.[479] The trigeminal ganglia contain a collection of neurons, the fibers of which transmit sensory information, including pain, from the blood vessels of the meninges, the layers around the brain as well as the scalp.[480] The brain itself does not contain receptors responsible for the transduction of painful stimuli. Not only did Dr. Moskowitz's work connect the vascular anatomy of the meninges and scalp with the neuroanatomy of headache pain, he also notes that the trigeminovascular neurons, the neurons innervating the meningeal blood vessels, contain substance P. Substance P is an 11 amino acid polypeptide that acts as a neurotransmitter-neuromodulator in the nervous system. In particular, substance P transmits pain impulses, dilates arteries of the pia (the inner lining of the brain), increases vascular permeability, and activates cells involved in the inflammatory response. These properties of substance P help explain the mechanism of sterile inflammation around blood vessels known to occur in migraine. Of interest is that capsaicin, the active ingredient in chile peppers (capsicum) reduces substance P.[481] It also reduces levels of calcitonin gene-related peptide (CGRP), a 37 amino acid peptide that is a very potent vasodilator and elevated during a migraine attack.[482]

The second seminal discovery, by researchers at Harvard, connects the CSD mentioned above with the pain of migraine related to activation of the trigeminal vascular system just discussed.[483] It is now proven by metabolic MRI and positron emission tomographic (PET) imaging that the CSD observed by Leao in rabbits occurs in humans as well. The CSD is a slowly progressing depolarization of glia and neurons on the cortical surface starting in the occipital lobe. As noted above, the meninges are innervated by small trigeminal nerve fibers that branch near small blood vessels. Bolay and the other researchers demonstrated in a rat migraine model that CSD triggers increased blood flow in pial (innermost meningeal layer) blood vessels, protein leakage in the dura mater, and activation of the trigeminal nucleus (the collection of nerve cell bodies of the trigeminal nerve). Edema was noted around some meningeal vessels. They observed an increase in a protein C-fos, responsible for gene transcription, in the cells of the trigeminal nucleus. This indicates activation of the trigeminal neurons responsible for transmission of pain impulses from the meninges. In essence, an electrical event in the cortex resulted in changes in the meningeal blood vessels and activation of the neuronal system responsible for transmitting pain impulses from the meninges to the central nervous system (CNS). We know that the trigeminal-vascular neurons contain vasoactive peptides such as substance P and possibly CRGP and neurokinin-1. In some way, the CSD triggers the release of these peptides that ultimately cause the vascular changes of migraine and contribute to the pain of migraine. Also of interest, studies suggest that CSD up-regulates other genes coding for COX-2, tumor necrosis factor-alpha (TNF-α), IL-1beta, and metalloproteinases, proteins discussed in other chapters in relation to chemical mediators of inflammation.[484] The metalloproteinases cause leakage of the blood brain-barrier allowing other inflammatory mediators to reach the dural perivascular trigeminal nerve terminals.

The preceding discussion helps explain the mechanism of individual migraine attacks and suggests certain herbs and nutrients, discussed below, to mitigate the process. The migraine syndrome though is more than isolated attacks of headache. In particular, it involves an increased susceptibility to a variety of conditions and stimuli that may trigger an attack. In addition, the recurrent attacks can transform into almost daily headaches, particularly with the influence of chronic opiate use or abuse. Transformed migraine is more difficult to overcome than the episodic discreet attacks of non-transformed migraine. All these factors suggest an alteration in the central processing of sensory stimuli and inhibition of the electrochemical cascade that triggers an individual attack. There is an increasing body of evidence to explain these aspects of migraine. One potent mechanism involves an alteration in the periaqueductal gray matter area in the brainstem. The periaqueductal gray matter is a columnar area of nerve cells, deep in the brainstem surrounding the aqueduct, the pathway of cerebrospinal fluid through the center of the brainstem at the base of the brain. This area gives rise to descending pathways that modulate the transmission of pain signals from the periphery, such as the pain sensitive structures in the head. In particular, this region modulates pain information transmitted through the trigeminal system discussed above. It also modulates other sensory input such as light and sound, known to be disinhibited in migraine. Finally, it is involved in the behavioral responses in opiate withdrawal.[485] Peripheral structures such as the trigeminovascular system discussed above do not have the capacity for complex information processing. That is the province of the CNS. Alterations in a central structure, such as the periaqueductal gray, can provide this capacity. Maintenance of normal iron levels in the periaqueductal gray is impaired in migraine patients providing evidence of dysfunction in migraine.[486]

Another major area of medical research impacting the understanding and treatment of migraine involves ion channels in cell membranes. Ion channels are pore forming membrane proteins, found in all cells, that provide for the controlled movement of ions into and out of cells. Defects in opening and closing a channel can result in human disease. Currently, mutations in sixty ion-channel genes are known to be associated with human disease.[487] The science of ion channels is increasingly complex. For our purposes we need to understand them as groups of subunit proteins embedded in the lipid bilayer that surrounds all cells. One subunit forms the pore while another is responsible for opening or closing the pore. Some channels are activated by changes in the voltage across the cell membrane while others respond to small molecules called ligands, either outside or inside the cell. Channels exist for multiple ions including chlorine, calcium, sodium, and potassium. The important inhibitory neurotransmitter gamma-aminobutyric acid (GABA) and glycine are ligands for chlorine channels whereas glutamate, an important excitatory neurotransmitter, is the ligand for calcium channels. There are also voltage-gated channels for sodium, potassium, and calcium. Voltage gated calcium channels are particularly important in seizures and pain disorders, including migraine. When the channel opens secondary to a change in its shape (or conformation) calcium flows into the cell. The calcium acts as a second messenger resulting in the release of neurotransmitters from the cell. In particular, glutamate and aspartate, excitatory neurotransmitters, are released. As discussed throughout *Integrated Medicine for Neurologic Disorders* glutamate, an essential neurotransmitter can be toxic when its concentration is excessive. By modulating the voltage dependent calcium channel, glutamate levels are reduced, alleviating its toxic effects. This appears to be the mechanism for the efficacy of the new drug pregabalin (Lyrica). It binds to a particular site called the alpha-2 delta subunit at the calcium channel and inhibits excessive influx of calcium.

One particular voltage-regulated calcium channel, the P/Q calcium channel, is genetically abnormal in a type of migraine called familial hemiplegic migraine. This autosomal dominant disorder involves migraine attacks associated with one-sided paralysis. The genetic mutation is known and involves the formation of abnormal proteins forming the alpha-1A subunit, the actual ion pore. The P/Q calcium channel is known to mediate release of excitatory neurotransmitters, although its function may be more complex than just mediating excitatory neurotransmitter release. Malfunction of this ion channel appears to result in a type of excitotoxicity causing hemiplegic migraine.[488] Some investigators have suggested that this particular genetic migraine disorder is only a specific example of a more general channelopathy occurring in more common migraine disorders. An English study in 2002 demonstrated that a disorder of the P/Q calcium channel in the peri-aqueductal gray alters pain modulation in the trigeminal pathways.[489] This seminal study, if replicated, may provide an important link between spreading cortical depression, the periaqueductal gray area and the changes in the trigeminovascular system, all occurring during the migraine attack. The periaqueductal area is a known modulator of pain transmitted to the CNS through the trigeminal cranial nerve system. Poor modulation of the voltage dependent calcium channel in the periaqueductal gray area may help explain the migraine patient's increased sensitivity to various stimuli that can precipitate a migraine attack.

The class of serotonin receptors appears more complex than the receptors noted above. Serotonin appears to activate second messengers which indirectly affect the function of ion channels. Second messengers are intracellular substances, created in response to a neurotransmitter or hormone acting on the cell membrane. They communicate between different parts of a cell and affect multiple intracellular activities. Calcium, nitric oxide, and cyclicAMP are examples. Calcium's role as a second messenger is discussed above.

Magnesium and Taurine

It has been known for some time that individuals with migraine have reduced levels of magnesium, both in the serum and intracellularly.[490,491,492] Up to 50% of patients have decreased magnesium during an acute attack. In addition, an intravenous infusion of magnesium can abort an acute attack and daily oral supplementation with magnesium can reduce the frequency of migraine attacks.[493] Magnesium appears to reduce migraine in several ways. It plays a significant role in inhibiting the flow of calcium into cells at an ion channel activated by glutamate. Glutamate acts on a specific receptor, the N-methyl d-aspartate (NMDA) receptor. When activated, the channel opens for several ions, potassium, sodium, and calcium. The influx of calcium and other ions may result in the release of more glutamate as well as substance P, a signaling molecule for pain. The magnesium ion blocks this channel outside the cell and needs to be expelled before it will open. Magnesium deficiency may disinhibit the NMDA receptor.

Magnesium appears to play a role in a superfamily of receptors called Transient Receptor Potential (TRP) ion channels. These channels appear to be unique, separate from the channels discussed above, although responsive to a wide variety of stimuli. They function in sensory receptors on the surface of the body, responsive to temperature, touch, pain, osmolarity, pheromones, vision, and probably hearing and smell. These stimuli modulate the anatomy of the receptors allowing an influx of ions, including calcium, resulting in transduction of information. They all share six loosely related families of proteins that transverse the cell membrane and contain a pore that allows influx of cations. Although research into TRP channels is in its early stages, it is known that magnesium is involved in the gating of some of these channels.[494] These channels exist in cells from yeast to nematodes to humans, and are essential to individual cellular function and protection as well as the function of multi-cellular organisms. Worms avoid noxious stimuli using TRP channels on the tip of neuronal processes in their noses. TRP channels guide mice to choose the appropriate gender in mating using pheromone sensitive TRP channels, and allow us to taste the various flavors such as sweet and bitter. They are found in the brain as well as multiple other organs including the heart, kidney, testis, lung, liver and so on. Not only are they found on sensory neurons but also in non-neuronal cells including vascular endothelial, epithelial, and smooth muscle cells. We introduce the reader to this family of ion channels with the expectation that they may play an increasing role in our understanding of reduced sensory thresholds in the migraine patient. Supplementation with magnesium may help restore this particular class of ion channels to a more normal level of functioning. Magnesium dosage varies considerably from 200-500mg/day. Magnesium loosens the bowels. This can be counteracted with calcium, 400mg/day, which has a binding effect.

An article in 1996 by McCarty suggests that magnesium and the amino acid taurine may act synergistically and magnesium taurate may be a better form of magnesium supplementation.[495] Taurine is an abundant acidic substance in animal tissues. It is related to the amino acids except that it contains a sulfonic acid group rather than a carboxylic acid group found in amino acids. One important physiologic function involves the binding of the amino group in taurine to the bile acids to form the bile salts important for the digestion of fats. Another essential function is its capacity to neutralize hypochlorous acid, a potent oxidizing compound in our body. The compound molecule is stable and acts as a buffer, mediating levels of hypochlorous acid and chlorine in our body. Also of interest is that taurine significantly elevated HDL levels in experimental animals and reduced atherosclerotic plaque formation by almost 30%.[496] Also of interest in atherosclerosis is the mild prolongation of the thrombin time by 9% and the inhibition of platelet aggregation by 10%.[497]

Pertinent to migraine is taurine's effects on glutamate, GABA, and intracellular calcium. Taurine appears to inhibit glutamate's effect of raising intracellular calcium. This was well established in studies at the University of Kansas in 2001.[498] Subsequent work demonstrated a reduction in calcium influx through specific voltage-gated calcium channels and the NMDA receptor calcium channel. Magnesium appeared essential for the taurine effect. The authors of the study conclude by saying: "We propose that taurine protects neurons against glutamate excitotoxicity by preventing glutamate-induced membrane depolarization, probably through its effect in opening chloride channels and, therefore, preventing the glutamate-induced increase in calcium influx and other downstream events."[499] This correlates with other studies demonstrating an agonist effect of taurine at GABA receptors, which are known to modulate the chloride channel. Of interest is that one article reports on taurine's ability to block the ability of beta-amyloid peptide induced glutamate excitotoxicity.[500] This has therapeutic implications for AD. The dosage of taurine varies from 500mg-4000mg/day. High dosages can cause loose stools and slightly increase gastric acid secretion.

Mitochondria in Migraine

The mitochondria are organelles, or subunits of cells, responsible for producing energy for cell function. An individual cell may have hundreds or thousands of mitochondria, each containing its own DNA, distinct from the DNA in the nucleus of the cell. Several metabolic cascades occur inside the mitochondria. Pyruvate, formed by the breakdown of glucose in the cytoplasm of the cell, is actively transported into the mitochondria where it is repeatedly changed in a circular metabolic enzymatic cascade called the

Kreb's cycle. Two molecules, NADH and FADH2, then enter a linear metabolic cascade of enzymes located on the inner lining of the mitochondria called the electron transport chain. If there is a problem in converting pyruvate via the Kreb's cycle (requiring oxygen), pyruvate is converted to lactate with substantially less energy production. The detailed chemistry inside the mitochondria is beyond the scope of this chapter. The basic chemistry is important in understanding the mitochondrial role in migraine and the use of CoQ10 and riboflavin in its treatment. There is a sequence of four large multiprotein complexes in the electron transport chain, three of which contain CoQ10. Electrons are donated from the molecules NADH and FADH2 to the first protein complex of the chain (NADH-CoQ reductase complex) and subsequently transported down the chain to the final repository of the electrons, water molecules. The energy released causes protons to be pumped from the inside of the mitochondria to area between the two membranes that contain the mitochondria. As the proton concentration builds up, the protons are transported back into the matrix (inside) of the mitochondria by an enzyme ATP synthase. This process is accompanied by the production of ATP from ADP and inorganic phosphate. This production of ATP is essential for the innumerable energy producing reactions in the body.

Any change in the normal molecular anatomy of the mitochondria can result in a loss of energy production. Different structural defects result in known mitochondrial disorders. These include progressive external opthalmoplegia, Leber hereditary optic neuropathy, mitochondrial encephalopathy, lactic acidosis, and stroke-like syndrome (MELAS), myoclonic epilepsy, MERRF (ragged-red fibers), and so on. Some disorders are clearly related to mutations in the mitochondrial DNA such as MELAS and MERRF. Migraine, on the other hand, appears to involve mitochondrial dysfunction without evidence for mitochondrial DNA mutations.[501] One simple study confirming mitochondrial dysfunction in migraine examined the relative levels of pyruvate and lactate in migraine, tension headache, and control patients. As noted above, pyruvate is normally converted in the Kreb's cycle to NADH and FADH2. This study found significantly increased levels of pyruvate and lactate in migraine patients suggesting a functional problem in mitochondrial energy metabolism.[502] More sophisticated measures of mitochondrial function involve magnetic resonance spectroscopy. This technique uses MRI instruments, but involves tuning the instrument to frequencies of specific atomic species such as phosphorus. Phosphorus binds with creatine, making the phosphorus available to ADP to form ATP. An early study in 1989 found a significant reduction in phosphocreatine and an increase in inorganic phosphate using magnetic resonance spectroscopy in migraine patients. The authors concluded that " ... energy phosphate metabolism ... appears disordered during a migraine attack."[503] Multiple subsequent studies from Italy have confirmed deficient or disorded energy metabolism in migraneurs.[504,505,506] Of interest is that a disordered energy metabolism with a reduction in ATP concentration may directly or indirectly affect the function of ion channels. The ion channels responsible for generating the transmembrane potential of about 70 millivolts rely on the availability of ATP. A reduction in ATP can affect the transmembrane potential, which in turn may affect the function of other channels, such as the calcium channels. Also of interest is a Russian article discussing Leao's CSD mentioned above. CSD might overwhelm local energy supplies. This in turn might directly or indirectly affect ion channel function as just discussed.[507]

Therapeutic measures to improve mitochondrial energy production in migraine involve studies with CoQ10 and riboflavin. As noted above CoQ10 is involved in three out of the four complexes in the electron transport chain. By increasing CoQ10 levels, it may be possible to improve cellular energy levels thereby making the brain more resistant to the migraine process. Several positive studies have been performed. An open label trial conducted at Thomas Jefferson University in Philadelphia on thirty-two patients showed significant benefit of 150mg/day.[508] A subsequent randomized controlled study in Zurich used 300mg/day on 42 migraine patients. A 50% decrease in attack frequency occurred in 47.6% of patients receiving CoQ10 and only in 14.4% in the placebo group.[509] Vitamin B2 (riboflavin) is an essential component of the molecule FADH2, which donates electrons in the electron transport chain. Similar to CoQ10, by increasing riboflavin levels with oral supplementation, it may be possible to increase cellular energy levels. A randomized controlled trial in Belgium utilized 400mg/day in fifty-five patients. A 50% improvement was seen in 59% of the riboflavin group and in only 15% of the placebo group.[510] A subsequent open study in Berlin utilized 400mg/day in an outpatient clinic. Headache frequency was significantly reduced from four days/month to two days/month and abortive drug usage declined from 7units/month to 4.5units/month. The authors conclude that: "In line with previous studies our findings show that riboflavin is a safe and well-tolerated alternative in migraine prophylaxis."[511]

Two other important mitochondrial nutrients are acetylcarnitine and alpha-lipoic acid (ALA). Acetylcarnitine is synthesized in the body by the enzyme ALC-transferase. The molecule serves a number of important functions. It facilitates the transport of acetyl CoA into the mitochondria as fuel for the citric acid cycle discussed above. It also combines with fatty acids for transport into the mitochondria. The fatty acids are metabolized by beta-oxidation yielding NADH and FADH2, substrates for the electron transport chain. Another benefit of supplementation is the increase of substrate (acetylcarnitine) for the ALC-transferase enzyme. As we age, oxidative damage to enzymes such as ALC-transferase reduces binding to its substrate. By increasing the amount of substrate we can increase the speed of the chemical reaction, ultimately improving mitochondrial function.[512] These are several ways in which acetylcarnitine promotes mitochondrial energy production. ALA is an important antioxidant discussed at length in other chapters. In terms of mitochondrial function, it serves as a coenzyme in the Kreb's cycle (also known as the citric acid cycle). It also raises the level of CoQ10, an essential nutrient in the electron transport chain, and levels of glutathione (GSH), the ultimate antioxidant in the mitochondria. A study in 2002 demonstrated that supplementation with acetyl-carnitine and ALA help restore mitochondrial structure and function.[513] A reasonable starting dosage of acetylcarnitine is 500mg twice/day and of ALA, 300mg/day of the sustained release formulation.

Herbs in migraine: The traditional, primary herbs for migraine are feverfew and butterbur. Feverfew, a name derived from the Latin word *febrifuge*, or fever reducing, has been part of the European herbal tradition for centuries. Used for fevers, arthritis, migraine, and a number of other indications, feverfew has anti-inflammatory properties. An early study in 1982 demonstrated inhibition of platelet phospholipase by feverfew.[514] The enzyme phospholipase releases arachidonic acid from membrane phospholipids resulting in pro-inflammatory prostaglandins. Feverfew's inhibition of phospholipase results in reduced proinflammatory prostaglandins. A more recent study from Yale reported on a study of parthenolide, a sesquiterpene lactone, the active ingredient of feverfew. Parthenolide was found to bind to and inhibit the molecule IkappaB kinase beta (IKKbeta).[515] IKKbeta is directly involved in allowing NF-kappa B to move from the cytoplasm into the nucleus initiating a cascade of pro-inflammatory events. NF-kappa B is an essential nuclear transcription factor found in all cell types. It turns on pro-inflammatory genes and is involved in cellular responses to stress, free radicals, and infection. A 2002 study at Harvard Medical School demonstrated increased activity of NF-kappa B in the initiation of migraine and its attenuation by parthenolide. Reduction in NF-kappa B levels preceded reduced inducible nitric oxide synthase levels in response to parthenolide.[516] The enzyme nitric oxide synthase produces nitric oxide, a highly diffusable gas involved in numerous biological processes including inflammation. Finally, a 2005 Italian study of parthenolide revealed, in an animal model, that it inhibited the activation of Fos by nitroglycerin in the trigeminal nucleus. As noted in the section above on Leao's spreading depression, Fos, or C-Fos, is a transcriptional protein in the trigeminal nucleus. Its presence indicates activation of neurons in the trigeminal nucleus responsible for transmission of pain signals from the meninges. Parthenolide also reduced activation of nuclear factor-kappaB in their study.[517]

Although a *Cochrane Database* review of feverfew trials found insufficient evidence for prophylactic efficacy,[518] several well-conducted trials did show significantly positive results. A German randomized, double-blind, placebo controlled study of 170 patients in 2005 was positive. The migraine frequency decreased almost in half in the experimental group.[519] Two older British studies also showed positive results for feverfew, both being double-blind, placebo controlled studies.[520,521] A study in 2003 established that parthenolide is effectively absorbed through the intestinal mucosa.[522] The cause for negative studies may relate to variable amounts of parthenolide in commercial products. A British study in 1992 demonstrated that the parthenolide content of products declined during storage and that products varied widely in their parthenolide content. Some products had no detectable parthenolide content.[523] Based on the evidence discussed above, an adequate, standardized parthenolide content is essential for the efficacy of a feverfew product. Dosage of feverfew, standardized to 1.2% parthenolide is 80-240mg twice/day.

Another herb that has efficacy in migraine is butterbur (Petasites hybridus). It is a perennial shrub that has been used for centuries for inflammatory disorders, including the plague, fever, cough, asthma, and skin wounds. Butterbur appears to have at least two anti-inflammatory mechanisms of actions. It is a selective COX-2 inhibitor. COX-2 is the enzyme responsible for the formation of inflammatory prostaglandins. In addition, butterbur extracts inhibit a mitogen-activated protein kinase (MAPK) named p42/44 MAPK. Protein kinase enzymes modify other proteins by phosphorylation, the addition of phosphate groups. They serve important modulatory functions in cells since up to 30% of all proteins can be modified by protein kinases. In particular, protein kinases affect the transmission of signals or information in cells including the regulation of gene function. The p42/44 MAPK is involved in an enzymatic cascade that affects gene transcription of inducible nitric oxide synthesis and COX-2. This may be how butterbur down-regulates COX-2.[524,525] As noted above, since nitric oxide may play a role in causing migraine, down-regulation of the gene responsible for the enzyme leading to its formation may be another pathway for the beneficial effect of butterbur. Finally, there are studies on another species of butterbur that demonstrate the inhibition of calcium channels.[526,527,528]

At least three studies have demonstrated a prophylactic effect of butterbur in migraine. All were randomized and placebo controlled, and one was double blind. The butterbur was well tolerated and all three studies show significant benefit of butterbur. Dosage was 50-75mg twice/day.[529,530,531]

Summary

Based on the information presented above, the following nutrients and herbs are recommended in migraine. As with all other maladies, every migraineur is different and requires individualized therapy. In particular, transformed migraine, the transformation of periodic migraine attacks to daily headaches, usually in the presence of excessive over-the-counter medications, requires very careful monitoring. Medical supervision is recommended. Scientific studies demonstrate metabolic changes in transformed migraine that are not present in non-transformed migraine.

Nutrients: Magnesium is essential with doses from 200mg twice/day up to 400-500mg twice/day depending upon GI tolerance. Taurine dosages range from 500- 4000mg/day in two divided dosages. Magnesium taurate may be an efficient way of supplementing with both nutrients. Dosages of CoQ10 vary from 30mg to several hundred mg/day. CoQ10 is a very safe nutrient but high quality, high dosage CoQ10 can be expensive. The standard riboflavin dosage is 400mg/day. Other mitochondrial nutrients that may be helpful include acetylcarnitine 500mg twice/day and ALA 300mg/day of a sustained release form.

Herbs: The dosage of feverfew is 80-240mg twice/day of a product standardized to 1.2% parthenolide content. The dosage of butterbur is 50-75mg twice/day.

Chapter Five Supplement Chart

Supplement	Dose	Frequency	Instructions
Acetylcarnitine	500mg	Twice/day	
Alpha-lipoic acid (ALA)	300mg	Day	Sustained release form
Butterbur	50-175mg	Twice/day	
CoQ10	30-150mg	Twice/day	
Feverfew	80-240mg	Twice/day	Standardized to 1.2% parthenolide
Magnesium	200-500mg	Twice/day	
Riboflavin	400mg	Day	
Taurine	500-4000mg	Day	Two divided dosages

Chapter Six

Seizure Disorders

In the U.S, recurrent seizures (epilepsy) occur in about 1% of individuals by the age of twenty.[532] It is estimated that fifty million individuals suffer from epilepsy worldwide, with the majority starting in childhood. Not only does the occurrence of seizures have a major impact on the quality of life of the individual, but the medications have both short- and long-term side effects. Control of seizures depends upon the seizure type and other factors specific to the individual. For some seizure types, up to 38% can be completely refractory to medications.[533] Additional medication may help reduce this figure, but each additional medicine brings diminishing returns and increased side effects. Based on the physiology of seizures, the addition of selected herbs and nutrients may help control seizures and make possible the reduction of medication dosages.

A limited discussion of the nature of epilepsy will be helpful in understanding the role of clinical supplementation (the use of herbs and nutrients). There are various classifications of seizures. The most commonly used is that proposed by the Commission on Classification and Terminology of the International League Against Epilepsy in 1981. Seizures can be divided into generalized, partial, or belonging to neither of these two groups. Generalized seizures can involve a convulsion (grand mal seizure) or a brief loss of consciousness (petit mal or absence seizure). They arise from the brain as a whole, usually without any warning, or aura. Generalized seizures tend to have a hereditary component in their causation. Partial seizures arise from a part of the brain, usually a small epileptic focus. In adults, this focus is most commonly in the temporal lobe, in particular the inner or mesial aspect of the temporal lobe. The structures in the mesial temporal lobe include the hippocampus, amygdala, and parahippocampal gyrus. The most common seizure type in adults is partial seizure arising from the temporal lobe.

Partial seizures may include loss of consciousness (complex partial seizures) or occur without loss of conscious (simple partial seizures). If the seizure spreads beyond the temporal lobe, it may become convulsive (secondary generalization). Because the temporal lobes integrate the whole spectrum of sensory information, seizures originating in the temporal lobe may involve sensations of smell, taste, visual imagery, and vertigo as well as specific memories or transient disorders of memory such as déjà vu, or jamais vu (strangeness of an otherwise familiar setting). Partial seizures tend to have a warning or aura (actually the beginning of the seizure).

The third type of seizure disorder is much less common. The seizure may involve jerks of the limbs (myoclonus) or seizures secondary to special stimuli such as a strobe light or even specific pieces of music. In childhood, seizure may occur with high fever (febrile seizures). Non-epileptic seizures can also occur, called pseudo seizures or hysterical seizures. Rather than a consequence of an abnormal electrical discharge from the cortex of the brain, pseudoseizures are psychogenic, driven perhaps by the subconscious mind of the individual.

Epileptic seizures result from a sudden electrical discharge of a localized group of abnormally excitable neurons or a bilateral network of excitable neurons possibly involving both the cortex and subcortical gray matter areas. Contributing factors may involve excessive activity of pathways involving the excitatory neurotransmitter glutamate or reduced activity in pathways involving the inhibitory transmitter gamma-aminobutyric acid (GABA). Reduced levels of the decarboxylated amino acid taurine or increased levels of glycine may be present. Increased sensitivity to the neurotransmitter acetylcholine may play a role and there may be inherited or non-genetic abnormalities in ion channels, particularly calcium channels.[534] These physiological mechanisms form the basis for the following discussion regarding the optimal use of herbs and nutrients to help mitigate the occurrence of seizures.

Anticonvulsant medications have multiple mechanisms of action, related to the neurotransmitter and ion channel abnormalities noted above. The sodium channel is voltage gated, meaning it is opened by changes in the transmembrane potential near the channel. When many sodium channels are grouped together, activation causes a large influx of sodium that depolarizes the cell membrane resulting in an action potential, the electrical potential that propagates rapidly down nerve fibers. Several epilepsy syndromes, including myoclonic epilepsy and inherited febrile seizures are related to inherited abnormalities in the sodium channel. Inhibition of the sodium channel is the primary antiseizure mechanism of Tegretol and Dilantin (phenytoin). Activation of the GABA receptor, the receptor for the inhibitory neurotransmitter GABA noted above, occurs with the use of phenobarbital, valproate (Depakote), and benzodiazepines

(Valium, Klonopin, Xanax, etc.). Another common antiseizure mechanism is inhibition of the receptor for glutamate, the main excitatory neurotransmitter in the brain. The anticonvulsants felbamate, phenobarbital, topiramate, zonisamide, lamotrigine, and valproic acid all inhibit the glutamate receptor. A new, novel mechanism of antiseizure medication is binding to a protein subunit on presynaptic calcium channels. Reduction of pre-synaptic calcium influx reduces release of glutamate, the excitatory neurotransmitter. Neurontin (gabapentin) and pregabalin (Lyrica) both appear to have this mechanism of action. Voltage-gated calcium channels are located presynaptically, the influx of calcium causing neurotransmitter release into the synapse. Abnormalities in the T-type channel cause juvenile myoclonic epilepsy and absence (petit mal) seizures. An old antiseizure drug, ethosuximide, appears to inhibit these specific channels in the thalamus.[535] The calcium channel blockers used for high blood pressure inhibit other types of calcium channels. Voltage gated potassium channels are also subject to genetic defects resulting in benign neonatal epilepsy. A new anticonvulsant, retigabine, currently in development, inhibits this channel.

GABA: The amino acid gamma-aminobutyric acid (GABA) is the main inhibitory neurotransmitter in the brain. In fact, GABA is the transmitter for 20-50% of all synapses in the central nervous system (CNS). Classically, GABA receptors are divided into A, B, and C, although C now appears to be a variant of A. The GABA A receptor controls a chloride channel and is the main type in the CNS. The influx of chloride hyperpolarizes the cell membrane. The anticonvulsants phenobarbital and sodium valproate enhance the inhibition of GABA, the latter through the upregulation of GABA metabolism.[536] The GABA receptor is unique in the variety of ligands (ions, atoms or molecules) that can bind to the receptor. These include anaesthetics, benzodiazepines (Valium, Xanax), and even pesticides. Of interest is that benzodiazepines change the shape of the receptor, making it more sensitive to the available GABA.[537]

Multiple studies report an association of seizures with reduced brain GABA levels. The relationship is somewhat complex and varies with treatment of the seizure disorders. An early study in 1979 demonstrated reduced cerebrospinal fluid GABA levels in twenty-one medicated patients with intractable seizures and also noted a greater reduction in patients with tonic-clonic and complex partial seizures than in those with simple partial seizures.[538] A Japanese study in 1985 demonstrated reduced GABA levels in patients with daily partial complex seizures and status epilepticus.[539] The most definitive study, reported from Yale University in 1996, measured in vivo GABA levels using 1H spectroscopy using a 2.1 Tesla magnetic resonance imager-spectrometer. Patients with complex partial seizures had significantly lower GABA levels than controls, with a correlation between low GABA levels and recent seizures. Patients who had a seizure within a day of testing had lower GABA levels than those who had no seizures within the past five years.[540]

GABA is the product of glutamic acid via the enzyme L-glutamic acid decarboxylase (GAD). Pyridoxal phosphate (vitamin B6) is an essential co-factor. GABA is metabolized by GABA transaminase, which also requires pyridoxal phosphate. The product of this reaction, succinic semialdehyde (SSAD) is converted by SSAD dehydrogenase to succinic acid. Of interest is that a negative feedback exists between succinic acid and glutamic acid decarboxylase, the formative enzyme of GABA. If GABA is reduced, GAD is up-regulated to form more GABA. An anticonvulsant, valproate acid, blocks SSAD dehydrogenase thereby decreasing succinic acid levels and up-regulating GAD to form more GABA. Another anticonvulsant, Vigabatrin, inhibits GABA transaminase, thereby increasing GABA levels. Gabrene (progabide) is an anticonvulsant that is converted to GABA in the body, thereby increasing activation at the GABA receptor. As discussed below, the amino acid taurine (lacking a carboxyl group) inhibits GABA transaminase, thereby increasing GABA levels. Finally, orally administered GABA is transported across the gut wall confirming its potential use as an adjunct in seizure control.[541]

As with other neurotransmitters, GABA has reuptake mechanisms, returning the molecule to the presynaptic neuron after it has been secreted into the synapse as a neurotransmitter. Reuptake into glial cells also occurs. There are four GABA transporters, GAT-1, GAT-2, GAT-3, and BGT-1. Although the accepted wisdom is that GABA has little if any ability to cross the blood-brain barrier, anecdotal experience and multiple studies suggest otherwise. Tight regulation of GABA influx from the blood is understandable to maintain tight control of CNS levels, particularly given the high prevalence of GABA synapses. In 1998, a Chinese study demonstrated both low and high affinity GABA transporters in cultured brain capillary cells.[542] A subsequent Chinese study in 1999 demonstrated the probable presence of the low affinity GABA transporter on the luminal surface of the capillaries and the high-affinity GABA transporter on the antiluminal surface.[543] Finally, a study in Japan in 2001 provided evidence for the GAT2/BGT-1 GABA transporter in blood-brain barrier cells. To quote: "These results are evidence that GAT2/BGT-1 is expressed at the BBB [blood-brain barrier] and is involved in GABA transport across the BBB."[544] Although these studies do not specify the directionality of GABA transport, two additional studies suggest blood to brain influx of GABA. Two Italian studies in 1992 reported on the influx of radio labeled GABA into the brain after intraperitoneal injection in rats. The radio labeled GABA entered the brain after a few minutes. At thirty minutes, 7% of the GABA in nerve endings was the exogenous radio labeled GABA.[545] A subsequent Italian study demonstrated that phosphatidylserine increased the blood-brain influx of GABA and accumulation into synaptosomes of the nerve endings.[546] In addition, transport into the blood stream from the gut does occur.[547] These studies support the use of supplementary oral GABA in a clinical protocol for seizure control. Depending upon capsule dosage, 500-1500mg twice/day is recommended, starting with only one dose, taken at bedtime. Higher dosages can be considered depending upon clinical response. Additional use of phosphatidylserine is recommended based on the Italian study noted above to enhance GABA influx from the blood into the brain. Recommended phosphatidylserine dosage is 100-150mg twice/day. The use of taurine and branched chain amino acids on GABA activity and glutamate metabolism is discussed below.

Glutamate, an amino acid, is the main excitatory neurotransmitter in the CNS. It is released from pre-synaptic neurons to act on multiple receptor types, including the NMDA, kainite, AMPA, and the non-ionic or metabotropic receptors. It actually is the amino acid glutamic acid that is ionized at the body's pH. There are multiple synthetic pathways for glutamic acid in the body. It may be derived from glutamine, a similar molecule except for an amine group instead of the hydroxyl group in glutamic acid. It can also be derived from alpha-ketoglutarate, a component of the Kreb's acid cycle, an important cyclic metabolic pathway related to the metabolism of carbohydrates. As noted above, glutamate is metabolized to GABA by GAD using pyridoxal phosphate as a co-factor. Thus, the principal excitatory neurotransmitter is metabolized to the main inhibitory one in one enzymatic step. Glutamate can be recycled to GABA by way of the Kreb's cycle mentioned above. The biochemical literature suggests that glutamic acid decarboxylase is essentially irreversible with little or no glutamate formed directly from GABA.[548] It is curious that the main inhibitory neurotransmitter is one irreversible metabolic step from the main excitatory neurotransmitter, glutamate. The irreversible metabolic step may provide protection against excess glutamate levels. The glutamate system is essential for learning and memory. The NMDA receptor is most important in the learning process, or encoding. The metabotropic receptors appear more involved in the modulation of consolidation or recall of memories.[549] GABA, in addition to a general inhibitory function, also appears involved in a particular type of learning, internal inhibition. Internal inhibition refers to the learned capacity to inhibit behavior that may result in pain. This information derives from conditioning experiments with animals.[550,551] The juxtaposition metabolically of glutamate and GABA may relate, in part, to the positive learning related to glutamate and the inhibitory learning related to GABA. The metabolic proximity also suggests an on-off switch. Of interest is that approximately 90% of cortical synapses are either GABA or glutamate synapses and excitatory synapses outnumber inhibitory synapses by about 5 to 1.[552]

Similar to GABA, glutamate is transported across membranes by transport molecules. These transporters are responsible for the reuptake of glutamate from the synaptic cleft, preventing excess levels and excitoxicity. There are five known transporters, called excitatory amino acid transporters (EAATs 1-5) which depend upon the electrochemical gradient of sodium and potassium. Vesicular glutamate transporters (VGLUTs 1-3), another type, are independent of sodium gradients and pack glutamate into presynaptic vesicles for subsequent release as a neurotransmitter. EAATs have 100-1000 times the affinity for glutamate as the VGLUTs. In addition to their presence in neurons and glial cells, the transporters provide active transport across the blood-brain barrier. There is evidence that diminished EAAT2 is associated with neurodegenerative disorders and overactivity of the transporters may be involved in schizophrenia. Pertinent to our discussion of seizures, experimental and human studies point to glutamate transporter abnormalities in epilepsy.[553] Glutamate modification with supplements is discussed below.

Taurine: Taurine is a small molecule with an amino group and a sulfur moiety but lacking the carboxyl group found in amino acids. It is pervasive in the animal and plant kingdoms but found in higher amounts in animals. Although manufactured from cysteine in the liver, taurine is notably reduced in vegans, possibly related to reduced taurine levels in plants. It has a number of important physiologic functions including a role in the formation of bile salts, osmoregulation and retinal function. Taurine is known to protect cultured neurons against glutamate excitotoxicity. This appears to occur through a reduction of the glutamate induced increase of intracellular calcium.[554] A recent study demonstrated taurine's inhibitory role in calcium influx through different calcium channels (L, P/Q, N-type voltage gated calcium channels and NMDA receptor calcium channels).[555] Taurine also appears to inhibit GABA transaminase, the enzyme that degrades GABA.[556]

Taurine levels appear to play a role in seizure disorders. Evidence comes from multiple sources including a recent Finnish study of amino acid levels in plasma and CSF (cerebrospinal fluid) after acute seizures. The only amino acid decreased in the CSF after seizures was taurine while the plasma demonstrated an increase in glutamate and aspartate, two excitatory amino acids.[557] Another interesting Swedish paper reported on the alteration of amino acids in the CSF in children on the ketogenic diet. The ketogenic diet is a very high fat diet (88% fat) producing a state of ketosis. Although known to reduce seizures, particularly in children, the mechanism has been unclear. The Swedish study demonstrated a statistically significant increase in GABA and taurine along with several other amino acids in children on the diet. Glutamate levels remained unchanged. GABA levels apparently correlated most significantly with response rate to the diet.[558] Finally, a 2003 study at the City University of New York demonstrated that taurine resulted in a significant reduction in seizures, mortality, and hippocampal neuronal apoptosis in mice injected with kainic acid. Kainic acid is a glutamate agonist and causes convulsions in rodents. The subcutaneous injection of taurine prior to the injection of kainic acid resulted in the beneficial effects noted above.[559]

Clinical studies with taurine in epilepsy are limited. Two studies suggest an initial response with gradual loss of effect. An Italian study in 1975 in what appears to be moderately severe epileptics revealed a therapeutic effect for about one month with return to baseline in two months.[560] A German study in 1977, again in refractory patients, showed a therapeutic effect lasting only for several weeks.[561] By definition, refractory patients tend not to respond to any therapeutic measures. A transient response suggests a therapeutic benefit gradually overwhelmed by pro-convulsive factors in this particular subset of patients. In addition, taurine was given alone. It is possible that a synergistic effect with multiple supplements may have resulted in a sustained benefit even in this problematic group of patients.

The foregoing information suggests a possible beneficial effect for oral taurine supplementation in seizure disorders.

Oral absorption of taurine is established[562] as is transport across the blood-brain barrier.[563] The latter study revealed reduced transport with higher CNS taurine levels and the presence of beta-alanine and increased transport with the presence of tumor necrosis factor-alpha (TNF-α) and hypertonic conditions. A study at the University of Michigan in 1995 demonstrated a natural tendency for a stable taurine influx rate into the CNS in the presence of increased plasma taurine or states of increased or decreased osmolarity.[564] Unfortunately, clinical information regarding blood to brain influx of taurine in general, and in epileptic states is limited. Taken as a whole, the studies noted above suggest deficient brain taurine levels in the presence of seizures, and a probable increased influx from blood to brain of taurine with supplementation under these circumstances. Given its safety and probable benefit, taurine supplementation is suggested in patients with seizures. Taurine dosage is up to 500mg-2gm twice/day on an empty stomach. A side effect at higher dosages is diarrhea.

Magnesium: Magnesium is an essential, primarily intracellular, macronutrient in the human body. It is an essential co-factor in numerous enzymatic reactions as well as in the formation of ATP, the denomination of energy utilized in all energy requiring enzymatic reactions. Magnesium also modulates the ion channel of the NMDA receptor, the receptor upon which the excitatory amino acid glutamate acts. Reduced magnesium levels increase the excitoxicity related to glutamate. The use of magnesium sulfate in pre-eclampsia to prevent seizures is well established. In addition, multiple studies demonstrate reduced magnesium levels in the serum and cerebrospinal fluid of epileptic patients[565,566,567] Studies also describe the occurrence of seizures in states of low magnesium.[568,569] In addition, magnesium can reduce seizure occurrence secondary to experimental neurotoxicity in animals.[570,571] In fact, one study demonstrated better efficacy of magnesium versus phenytoin in NMDA induced seizures in rats.[572] Unfortunately, even with multiple factors supporting the anticonvulsant properties of magnesium, an extensive literature search has not revealed a single study using magnesium supplementation in individuals with epilepsy. This is unfortunate for individuals with recurrent seizures, particularly given the extreme safety of supplemental magnesium. Based upon the information presented above, we recommend the use of a chelated magnesium supplement to reduce seizure potential. Dosage is 100-300mg twice/day. Higher dosages may cause diarrhea which can be counteracted by adding calcium to the magnesium supplementation.

Skullcap: A woodland herb, skullcap (*Scutellaria lateriflora*) is native to North America. It has been used herbally in England and in North America, including use by the Cherokee Indians. In the 1800s and early 1900s skullcap was used in North America by the Eclectics, herbalists who approached herbal medicine quantitatively with measurements and extracts and who played a role in the early pharmaceutical industry. It has been used variably for rabies (called Mad Dog herb), anxiety, depression, insomnia, and headache. Traditionally it has also been used for epilepsy, although scientific validation is quite limited. There is one 2004 Canadian study in rats, revealing an antiepileptic effect of skullcap in seizures induced by lithium and pilocarpine.[573] Dosage of a 1:2 strength tincture is 1-3 dropperfuls three times/day.

Bacopa: Bacopa monnieri is a perennial, creeping herb with relatively thick, succulent leaves. It grows in marshy areas in India, Nepal, Sri Lanka, China, and Taiwan, as well as the southern states of the U.S. Since 500 C.E. it has been an important nervine in Ayurvedic medicine, the indigenous medicine of India dating back 5,000 years. It is part of a class of herbs called medhya rasayana, Sanskrit for rejuvenation of cognition.[574] A significant amount of research on the neurologic benefits of bacopa can be found in Medline. This includes a 2006 study from Texas A&M University showing reduced levels of amyloid in mice exposed to bacopa.[575] This study used a transgenic variety of mice, PSAPP mice, that overexpressed amyloid precursor protein. Bacopa has significant CNS antioxidant capacity[576] and adaptogenic qualities,[577] the ability to reverse the biochemical markers of stress. Reports indicate that Bacopa reduces the production of reactive oxygen species, DNA fragmentation, and increases metabolic enzymes and processes necessary for handling stress.[578,579,580] This finding is important given the known increased oxidative stress in epileptic states. Studies also report its value in improving cognitive function.[581] These properties of Bacopa recommend its consideration for use in the neurodegenerative disorders discussed in other chapters of this book. Direct experimental evidence for a salutary influence of Bacopa in seizures is limited. A 2004 study demonstrated an anticonvulsant effect of an Ayurvedic formulation Unmadnashak Ghrita. This formulation contains Bacopa along with three other herbs.[582] There is another 2000 study showing that Bacopa reduced the cognitive side effects of phenytoin in animals.[583] Finally, there is reference to a 1966 study on the antiseizure properties of Bacopa, although this article is not available.[584] Based on its antioxidant, adaptogenic, and cognitive enhancing qualities as well as its traditional use and limited experimental evidence for its use in epilepsy, we recommend its consideration in individuals with seizures. Dosage forBacopa is 100mg twice/day of a product standardized to bacosides. Take Bacopa with meals.

Valerian: Several experimental studies support the potential antiseizure properties of *Valeriana alliariifolia* (valerian), an herb used since the time of Galen in ancient Greece. Aqueous extracts of valerian inhibit the uptake, and stimulate the release of, GABA from synaptosomes in isolated rat brain cortex.[585] Another study confirmed binding of extracts of valerian to the GABA receptor[586] and valerian appears to inhibit GABA catabolism.[587] Finally, a Russian study in 1987 refers to the anticonvulsant effects of valepotriates isolated from valerian.[588] The GABA-ergic properties and limited data on anticonvulsant effects suggest the use of valerian in seizure disorders. Dosage is 200-600mg two-three times/day.

Peony root: Peonies are classified in Ranunculaceae family, similar to buttercups. They are tall plants with showy flowers. They are common to Japan and China and occur in hundreds of hybrid varieties. White Peony, or Paeonia lactiflora (alba) is the variety most common in herbal medicine. A number of recent studies have been conducted on the anticonvulsant properties of peony root. A Japanese study in 1991 demonstrated evidence for reduced cellular influx of calcium.[589] Calcium influx can result in neuronal release of excitatory neurotransmitters such as glutamate. In 2004, another Japanese study showed that peony root increased expression of the gene A20, a gene that inhibits apoptosis of neurons.[590] It appears to inhibit TNF activation of the pro-inflammatory transcription factor NF-kappa B. This suggests applications in the neurodegenerative disorders discussed in other chapters of the book. Most telling is a 2006 Japanese study revealing the mechanism of peony's inhibiting of bursting activity, a state of high frequency electrical discharge of a neuron. Peony appears to inhibit the calcium activation of the potassium influx current, required for generation of electrical discharges.[591] These studies are very promising for the use of peony root in seizure disorders. Dosage is one gm/day of herb in tea. The alcohol extract dosage is unclear and depends upon the tincture concentration. For a 1:1 concentration, consider 1-5 ml (one teaspoon) twice/day.

Summary

Epilepsy (recurrent seizures) requires ongoing medical care. There is no evidence that seizures can be completely controlled with the use of herbs and nutrients without medication. On the other hand, as discussed above, herbs and nutrients may well help control seizures, allow reduction of medication dosage, and provide neuroprotection in the presence of seizures. As with all disorders, any seizure patient interested in the use of supplements requires individual evaluation for the best choice of supplements as well as ongoing supervision. The following summarizes the use of herbs and nutrients in seizure disorders.

GABA: GABA is the main inhibitory amino acid neurotransmitter in the brain. Clinical experience and review of the available literature suggest it does cross the blood-brain barrier, contrary to the commonly held opinion that it does not. GABA is relatively safe and generally inexpensive. It can be sedative early on so the dose should be gradually titrated. Starting at 500-750mg at bedtime, the individual may slowly increase the dose as high as 1500mg twice/day. As noted above, phosphatidylserine appears to help GABA cross the blood-brain barrier. Phosphatidylserine dosage is 100-150mg twice/day.

Taurine: Taurine is an amino acid minus the amino group and is pervasive in the body's metabolism. It inhibits the excitatory effects of glutamate and inhibits the enzyme that metabolizes GABA, the brain's main inhibitory neurotransmitter. Both these effects are important in controlling seizures. Starting at 500mg on an empty stomach at bedtime, the dosage can be increased slowly up to 2gm twice/day.

Magnesium: Magnesium is an essential mineral with numerous functions in the body's metabolism. Its value in seizures relates to its inhibitory role in the ion channel of the NMDA receptor, an important receptor for glutamate and the main excitatory neurotransmitter in the brain. In addition, magnesium levels tend to be reduced in individuals with seizures. A chelated (bound to amino acids) form of magnesium is recommended rather than an inorganic form such as magnesium oxide or carbonate. The organic chelated form is better absorbed and the amino acid may be beneficial as well. In fact, magnesium taurate is available providing both magnesium and taurine. Magnesium dosage varies from 100-300mg twice/day. At higher dosages, magnesium may cause diarrhea, which can be mitigated with the concurrent use of calcium at a similar dosage to the magnesium.

Herbs: Although a number of herbs have traditional usage in epilepsy, skullcap, bacopa, peony root, and valerian appear to have the most scientific support. Peony root, in particular, appears to inhibit calcium influx, an essential current for release of excitatory neurotransmitters. It also inhibits the gene essential for apoptosis and inhibits an important element of the metabolic cascade leading to inflammation. These latter properties suggest a role in neuroprotection. Finally, it appears to inhibit the high-frequency voltage discharge of neurons, a type of neuronal firing, that occurs in epilepsy. Bacopa appears to have neuroprotective properties, enhances cognition, and has traditional usage in epilepsy. For individuals with frequent seizures, neuroprotection is important to limit neuronal excitotoxicity and stress. Valerian, used for millennia, appears to have GABA enhancing properties, similar to a number of the pharmaceutical anticonvulsants. Smell and taste is a bit of an obstacle to the otherwise safe usage of this herb. Finally, skullcap is a traditional anticonvulsant herb with limited modern scientific study. The lack of evidence does not imply a lack of efficacy, and traditional usage is generally a good guide to an herb's indication in a clinical setting.

Herbs can be utilized as aqueous extractions (teas or decoctions), alcohol extractions (tinctures), encapsulated dried herb, or gaseous extractions yielding increased potency encapsulated powders. An advantage to tinctures is the capacity for blending a combination of extracts into a single tincture. All the herbs noted above come as tinctures, and can be mixed together into a single tincture. For high potency tinctures with a 1:1 or 1:2 ratio of herbal mg to alcohol ml, one or more teaspoons twice/day is recommended. Based on the evidence presented above, a higher proportion of peony root in the tincture is recommended.

Chapter Six Supplement Chart

Supplement	Dose	Frequency	Instructions
GABA	500-1500mg	Twice/day	Start with one dose only, taken at bedtime
Magnesium	100-300mg	Twice/day	
Phosphatidyl-serine	100-150mg	Twice/day	
Taurine	500mg-2gm	Twice/day	Empty stomach
1:1 or 1:2 Tinctures of peony root, bacopa, skullcap, & valerian	1tsp	Twice/day	Combine into one tincture with a higher proportion of peony root

Conclusion

By the time this book reaches publication science will have uncovered further mechanisms underlying the neurologic maladies from which we suffer. Currently, thousands of research papers are being published illuminating mechanisms of disease unheard of twenty-five years ago. These mechanisms include the role of the proteasome in cellular protein disposal, sirtuins in gene silencing, genetic alterations in neurodegenerative disorders, cellular signaling mechanisms and genetic and acquired disorders in ion channels. Complementing this will be new research on herbs and nutrients, mitigating the pathology engendered by these abnormal processes.

Archeological evidence suggests the medicinal use of herbs dating back 60,000 years, and adequate nutrition has always been essential for living organisms. A startling study, called the Kames Project, illuminates just how important nutrients are in preventing neurologic disease. This study is a collaborative project of the University of Washington and the immigrant Japanese-American community in Seattle. The study looks at various health issues of aging, particularly cognitive decline. A new paper from the Kames project, released in September 2006, reports the hazard ratios of individuals developing probable AD as a function of frequency of vegetable and/or fruit juice consumption. Those drinking juice three or more times per week had a 76% less likelihood of developing AD than those consuming juice less than one time weekly.[592] This figure is not the 30–40% benefit of a large number of drugs we use in these disorders, but a 76% reduction. It is unnecessary to analyze the nutrient and antioxidant components of vegetable or fruit juice to be impressed with the results of the Kames study. It points to the value of obtaining our nutrients from food, if possible. It also underscores the essential unitary nature of antioxidant systems. Outcome studies looking at the benefits of a single antioxidant, such as vitamin E, ignore the basic system biochemistry of antioxidants.

If the narrative of recent research has any predictive value, we believe that the commonly used supplements will continue to play a role in the treatment of neurologic disorders, given any new and novel mechanisms of disease uncovered through basic research. It is our hope that *Integrated Medicine for Neurologic Disorders* will provide both practitioners and patients alike an ongoing reference to help integrate herbs and nutrients into the care of individuals suffering from these disorders.

About the Authors

Sidney Kurn, M.D. has been practicing neurology since 1979. He has a strong interest in integrating alternative approaches to the treatment of neurologic disorders, adding acupuncture to his practice in 1994 and herbal medicine in 1996. Dr. Kurn's contribution to *Integrated Medicine for Neurologic Disorders* is based in a large part on his experience using various herbs and supplements in the disorders discussed in this book. He is also the cofounder of the herbal pharmacy Farmacopia located in Santa Rosa, California. Dr. Kurn is an Associate Clinical Professor at the University of California, San Francisco Medical Center and a member of the American Academy of Neurology as well as the American Academy of Medical Acupuncture.

Sheryl Shook, Ph.D. earned her doctorate in neuroscience from University of California, Davis. She has completed studies in herbal medicine and currently is an anatomy and physiology professor. Dr. Shook's strong desire to teach and empower others in their own healing has led to her co-authorship of this book. She lives in Davis, California, with her husband and daughter.

Epilogue

Neurodegenerative Disorders
and Multiple Sclerosis

In the short time since the writing of the foregoing chapters, research continues to bring new information about the mechanisms of these disorders and the potential benefits of various herbs and nutrients. The Introduction to *Integrated Medicine for Neurologic Disorders* hints at a framework for both the understanding and the supplemental treatment of the disorders considered neurodegenerative. It briefly summarizes four mechanisms: inflammation, oxidation, excitotoxicity, and environmental toxicity. It is increasingly evident that genetics also plays a role in all of these disorders. In Alzheimer's disease, abnormal alleles, or gene variants, in the Apolipoprotein E (APOE), amyloid precursor protein, and presenilin genes increase an individual's susceptibility to Alzheimer's Disease (AD). Similarly, nine genes, PARK 1-8 and PARK 10 play an etiologic role in Parkinson's disease (PD). It is well known that migraine has a familial tendency, and that one type, familial hemiplegic migraine, has a specific genetic variant resulting in an abnormal calcium ion pore protein. Although quite complex, certain genetic profiles appear to underlie the known familial tendency in multiple sclerosis (MS). One genetic predilection to MS involves the

Human Leukocyte Antigen (HLA) complex of genes on the 6th chromosome. Certain HLA alleles have a strong correlation with various measures of MS severity.[593] Also of interest is the discovery in 2007 of a strong correlation of a paraoxonase allele and the risk of MS. Mentioned in the Introduction in reference to atherosclerosis, this enzyme is involved in detoxification and free-radical scavenging. A study at the University of Messina in Italy found a strong correlation of a specific paraoxonase allele to the risk for developing MS.[594]

Another important factor in the emergence of a neurologic disorder is a nutrient deficiency or a combination of deficiencies. This is particularly salient in migraine and PD. Reports in 2006 and 2007 add a new dimension to the known vitamin D deficiency in MS. Experimental studies in vitamin D deficient mothers revealed dysregulation of multiple proteins and metabolic pathways in their offspring. These pathways included oxidative energy production (phosphorylation), redox balance, synaptic plasticity, and neurotransmission among other abnormalities. A correlation with mitochondrial dysfunction was also found. The dysregulated proteins and pathways appear to correlate with abnormalities found in MS.[595,596] This information may help elucidate the epidemiology of MS. MS incidence is known to increase with distance from the equator and decreasing sunlight exposure (lower vitamin D levels). Migration from northern to southern latitudes as a child confers the lower, southern incidence of MS on the migrating population whereas migration as an adult does not alter the higher incidence of the disease seen in northern latitudes. Vitamin D deficiency in the mothers appears to affect brain development, perhaps increasing susceptibility to MS. Moving to southern latitudes, with their increasing vitamin D levels, as a child may mitigate this effect.

Although too involved a subject for an epilogue, mention should be made of the interaction of the various disease risk factors noted above, including positive feedback among inflammation, oxidation, genetic variants, nutrient deficiencies, and xenobiosis. Historically we have viewed PD, AD, MS, and so on, as separate, distinct entities. Given similar underlying abnormal mechanisms, it is conceivable that each disease is simply a different pathogenic pathway, determined by the relative nature and magnitude of each component of the system. Not only does this unify our view of neurologic disorders but it supports and directs the use of various antioxidant, anti-inflammatory, and detoxifying supplements in any particular disorder.

Several studies also bring MS into the neurodegenerative framework. Although traditionally viewed as a primary demyelinating disorder, new research calls this view into question.[597] Axonal loss is now viewed as the major factor in irreversible disability, may begin at disease onset, and may be the principal factor in the progressive phase of the disease[598]. Questions remain whether axonal loss is secondary to the inflammation involving myelin or occurs secondarily to different albeit overlapping mechanisms. Axonal involvement may explain the relative lack of correlation between MRI images and clinical symptoms and signs. Of particular interest for us is the potential role of mitochondria in axonal degeneration, perhaps similar in some respects to its rather central role in PD. One interesting hypothesis involves the exhaustion of mitochondrial function in the long chronic phase of the disease.[599] Conduction along a demyelinated axon is difficult, with redistribution of sodium channels, essential elements in the transmission of the electric current along the fiber. More energy is required in this setting, supplied by mitochondria, the energy producing organelles in all cells. As discussed throughout the book, free radical production is unavoidable in mitochondrial energy production. Increased mitochondrial function yields increased free radicals and a consequent increase in oxidative damage to mitochondrial components. Loss of mitochondria ultimately leads to nerve cell death (apoptosis). The final common pathway of MS may be the same as that which occurs in the more commonly designated neurodegenerative disorders.[600]

Research reveals that the white matter, or myelin, in otherwise normal appearing areas of the brain in an MS patient is altered biochemically. Myelin basic protein (MBP), an important protein in myelin, has a significant increase in the amino acid citrulline compared to the white matter of individuals without MS. The increased citrulline occurs at the expense of arginine via an enzyme peptidyl arginine deiminase 2 (PAD 2). This change in amino acids apparently reduces the magnitude of positive charge of MBP and interferes with the protein's ability to interact with the lipid bilayer that composes myelin.[601] The same research group at the Hospital for Sick children in Toronto, Canada then discovered that the gene responsible for the enzyme PAD 2 is significantly more active. This increased activity is traced to a demethylation of the promoter portion of the gene, the portion of the gene that interacts with transcription factors (molecules that tell the gene to turn on production of its protein product). Methylation of a gene, the addition of a methyl group (a carbon attached to four hydrogens) turns off a gene. Demethylation, or loss of the methyl group, turns on the gene. This in turn appears related to an increase in an enzyme DNA demethylase, to twice normal levels.[602]

The research just discussed has a significant potential to impact MS theory. For many years, plaques, or volumes of demyelination in the brain has been the pathologic hallmark of MS. Axonal injury, mitochondrial dysfunction, and in particular, biochemical abnormalities in seemingly normal brain areas, moves our understanding of MS into a much wider, potentially more fruitful area of investigation. It also suggests the possible application of various neuroprotective nutrients discussed in the chapters on PD and AD, particularly in the progressive phase of the disease. Coenzyme Q10 (CoQ10) and acetylcarnitine provide mitochondrial support and Ginkgo biloba is protective of the energy producing enzymatic reactions in the mitochondria. Antioxidant protection is supported by alpha-lipoic acid (ALA), N-acetylcarnitine, and vitamins C and E. Excitotoxicity can be mitigated by magnesium, taurine, gamma-aminobutyric acid (GABA), and huperzine A. None of these nutrients is particularly immune-stimulating and should prove safe in MS.

Finally, the demethylation of the PAD 2 gene, resulting ultimately in changes in MBP, may respond to resveratrol. This polyphenol, found in the skin of grapes, is discussed at length in the chapter on PD. Of its many salutary properties, it appears to affect favorably the epigenetics of the organism. Epigenetics is the study of the chemical modification of DNA which leads to turning on and off genes. Breaking the DNA code, or learning the nucleotide sequence of our DNA, as monumental as it is, is only part of the puzzle. Knowing which genes are on or off is also essential. There are several epigenetic mechanisms, one of which (the methylation of the promoter region of a gene) is mentioned above. Not only is our epigenetics inherited, the epigenetic mechanisms age, losing their functional capacity. Excess protein production from demethylated genes is part of the aging phenomenon. Resveratrol can help restore this capacity through methylation of DNA[603] as well as tightening the proteins (called histones) wrapped around the DNA. It does this by increasing sirtuins, enzymes that remove chemical components called acetyl groups, from histones. Resveratrol may potentially improve MBP in patients with MS by down regulating the PAD 2 gene responsible for the enzyme that modifies normal MBP. Although this is hypothetical at this point, in the absence of scientific studies, resveratrol appears quite safe as a supplement. Dosages for the herbs and nutrients just noted may be found in the body of the book, particularly in the PD and AD chapters.

We hope that *Integrated Medicine for Neurologic Disorders* will help clear the way and, to some extent, empower the reader in the pursuit of his or her better health. Your health ultimately lies within you. Safe journey...

References

1. Dokmeci D. Ibuprofen and Alzheimer's disease. *Folia Med* (Plovdiv). 2004;46(2):5-10.

2. Swarnakar S, et al. Curcumin regulates expression and activity of matrix metalloproteinases-9 and -2 during prevention and healing of indomethacin-induced gastric ulcers. *J Biol Chem*. 2004 Dec 22; (Epub ahead of print).

3. Chainani-Wu N. Safety and anti-inflammatory activity of curcumin: a component of turmeric (Curcuma Longa). *J Altern Complement Med*. 2003 Feb;9(1):161-8.

4. Leu TH and Maa MC. The molecular mechanisms for the antitumorigenic effect of curcumin. *Curr Med Chem Anti-Canc Agents*. 2002 May;2(3):357-70.

5. Gilgun-Sherki Y, et al. The role of oxidative stress in the pathogenesis of multiple sclerosis: the need for effective antioxidant therapy. *J Neurol*. 2004 Mar;251 (3):261-8.

6. Veurink G, et al. Genetics, lifestyle and the roles of amyloid-beta and oxidative stress in Alzheimer's disease. *Ann Hum Biol*. 2003 Nov-Dec;30(6):639-67.

7. Madamanchi NR, et al. Oxidative stress in atherogenesis and arterial thrombosis: the disconnect between cellular studies and clinical outcomes. *J Thromb Haemost*. 2005 Feb;3(2):254-67.

8. Packer L, et al. Neuroprotection by the metabolic antioxidant alpha-lipoic acid. *Free Radic Biol Med*. 1997;22(1-2):359-78.

9. Packer L. Alpha-lipoic acid: a metabolic antioxidant which regulates NF-kappa-B signal transduction and protects against oxidative injury. *Drug Metab Rev*. 1998 May;30(2):245-75.

10. Blaylock RL. *Excitotoxins: The Taste that Kills*. Health Press. Santa Fe. New Mexico. 1997.

11. Meister B, et al. Neurotransmitters, neuropeptides and binding sites in the rat mediobasal hypothalamus: effects of monosodium glutamate (MSG) lesions. *Exp Brain Res.* 1989;76(2):343-68.

12. Hu L, et al. Exogenous glutamate enhances glutamate receptor subunit expression during selective neuronal injury in the ventral arcuate nucleus of postnatal mice. *Beuroendocrinology.* 1998 Aug;68 (2):77-88.

13. Olney JW, et al. Increasing brain tumor rates: is there a link to aspartame. *J Neuropathol Exp Neurol.* 1996 Nov;55(11):1115-23.

14. Junn E and Mouradian MM. Apoptotic signaling in dopamine-induced cell death: the role of oxidative stress, p38 mitogen-activated protein kinase, cytochrome c and caspases. *J Neurochem.* 2001 Jul;78(2):374-83.

15. Zhang J, et al. Secondary excitotoxicity contributes to dopamine-induced apoptosis of dopaminergic neuronal cultures. *Biochem Biophy Res Commun.* 1998 Jul 30;248(3):812-6.

16. Kostrzewa RM and Segura-Aguilar J. Novel mechanisms in the study of neurodegeneration and neuroprotection. A review. *Neurotox Res.* 2003;5(6):375-83.

17. Firestone JA, et al. Pesticides and risk of Parkinson disease: a population-based case-control study. *Arch Neurol.* 2005 Jan;62(1):91-5.

18. Koldkjaer OG, et al. Parkinson's disease among Inuit in Greenland: organochlorine as risk factors. *Int J Circumpolar Health.* 2004;63 Suppl 2:366-8.

19. Cory-Slechta DA, et al. Developmental pesticide exposure and the Parkinson's disease phenotype. *Birth Defects Res A Clin Mol Teratol.* 2005 Mar;73(3):136-9.

20. Snyder H and Wolozin B. Pathological proteins in Parkinson's disease: focus on the proteasome. *J Mol Neurosci.* 2004;24(3):425-42.

21. Corrigan FM, et al. Organochlorine insecticides in substantia nigra in Parkinson's disease. *J Toxicol Environ Health A.* 2000 Feb 25;59(4):229-34.

22. Fleming L, et al. Parkinson's disease and brain levels of organochlorine pesticides. *Ann Neurol.* 1994 Jul;36(1):100-3

23. Zhou Y, et al. Proteasomal inhibition induced by manganese ethylene-bis-dithiocarabamate: relevance to Parkinson's disease. *Neuroscience.* 2004;128(2):281-91.

24. Snyder H and Wolozin B. Pathological proteins in Parkinson's disease: focus on the proteasome. *J Mol Neurosci.* 2004;24(3):425-42.

25. Alam M and Schmidt WJ. Mitochondrial complex I inhibition depletes plasma testosterone in the rotenone model of Parkinson's disease. *Physiol Behav.* 2004 Dec 15;83(3):395-400.

26. Aviram M and Rosenblat M. Paraoxonases 1,2 and 3, oxidative stress, and macrophage foam cell formation during atherosclerosis development. *Free Radic Biol Med.* 2004 Nov 1;37(9):1304-16.

27. Mackness MI, et al. Low serum paraoxonase: a risk factor for atherosclerotic disease. *Chem Biol Interact.* 1999 May 14;119-120:389-97.

28. Baldi I, et al. Neurodegenerative diseases and exposure to pesticides in the elderly. *Am J Epidemiol.* 2003 Mar 1;157 (5) :409-14.

29. Baldi I, et al. Neuropsychological effects of long-term exposure to pesticides: results from the French Phytoner study. *Environ Health Perspect.* 2001 Aug;109(8):839-44.

30. Cooper GS, et al. Occupational exposure and autoimmune diseases. *Int Immunopharmacol.* 2002 Feb;2(2-3):303-13.

31. U.S. Geological Survey. Mercury in the environment. Available at: http://www.usgs.gov/themes/factsheet/146-00/. Accessed August,15, 2006.

32. Virtanen JK, et al. Mercury, fish oils, and risk of acute coronary events and cardiovascular disease, coronary heart disease, and all-cause mortality in men in eastern Finland. *Arterioscler Thromb Vasc Biol.* 2005 Jan;25(1):228-33. Epub 2004 Nov 11.

33. Foran SE, et al. Measurement of mercury levels in concentrated over-the-counter fish oil preparations: is fish oil healthier than fish. *Arch Pathol Lab Med.* 2003 Dec;127(12):1603-5.

34. Gorell JM, et al. Occupational metal exposure and the risk of Parkinson's disease. *Neuroepidemiology.* 1999;18(6):303-8.

35. Gorrell JM, et al. Occupational exposures to metals as risk factors for Parkinson's disease. *Neurology.* 1997 Mar;48(3):650-8.

36. Uversky VN, et al. Metal-triggered structural transformations, aggregation, and fibrillation of human alpha-synuclein. A possible molecular NK between Parkinson's disease and heavy metal exposure. *J Biol Chem.* 2001 Nov 23;276(47):44284-96. Epub 2001 Sep 11.

37. Waterman SJ, et al. Lead alters the immunodenicity of two neural proteins; a potential mechanism for the progression of lead-induced neurotoxicity. *Environ Health Perspect.* 1994 Dec;102(12):1052-6.

38. Bates MN, et al. Health effects of dental amalgam exposure: a retrospective cohort study. *Int J Epidemiol.* 2004 Aug; 33(4) :894-902. Epub 2004 May 20.

39. Mutter J, et al. (Amalgam risk assessment with coverage of references up to 2005). *Gesundheitswesen.* 2005 Mar;67(3):204-16.

40. Mutter J, et al. Alzheimer disease: mercury as pathogenetic factor and apolipoprotein E as a moderator. *Neuro endocrinol Lett.* 2004 Oct;25(5):331-9.

41. Martinelli Boneschi F, Rovaris M, Johnson KP, et al. Effects of glatiramer acetate on relapse rate and accumulated disability in multiple sclerosis: meta-analysis of three double-blind, randomized, placebo-controlled clinical trials. *Mult Scler.* 2003;9(4):349-355.

42. Murray M, Pizzorno J. Encyclopedia of Natural Medicine. Rocklin, California: Prima Publishing; 1998.

43. Lupton JR. Dietary reference intakes for trans fatty acids: National Academy Press; 2002.

44. Swank RL. Multiple sclerosis; a correlation of its incidence with dietary fat. *Am J Med Sci.* 1950;220(4):421-430.

45. Swank RL, Lerstad O, Strom A, Backer J. Multiple sclerosis in rural Norway its geographic and occupational incidence in relation to nutrition. *N Engl J Med.* 1952;246(19):722-728.

46. Esparza ML, Sasaki S, Kesteloot H. Nutrition, latitude, and multiple sclerosis mortality: an ecologic study. *Am J Epidemiol.* 1995;142(7):733-737.

47. Ben-Shlomo Y, Davey Smith G, Marmot MG. Dietary fat in the epidemiology of multiple sclerosis: has the situation been adequately assessed? *Neuroepidemiology.* 1992;11(4-6):214-225.

48. Sinclair HM. Deficiency of essential fatty acids and atherosclerosis, etcetera. *Lancet.* 1956;270(6919):381-383.

49. Tsang WM, Belin J, Monro JA, Smith AD, Thompson RH, Zilkha KJ. Relationship between plasma and lymphocyte linoleate in multiple sclerosis. *J Neurol Neurosurg Psychiatry.* 1976;39(8):767-771.

50. Dworkin RH, Bates D, Millar JH, Paty DW. Linoleic acid and multiple sclerosis: a reanalysis of three double-blind trials. *Neurology.* 1984;34(11):1441-1445.

51. Nordvik I, Myhr KM, Nyland H, Bjerve KS. Effect of dietary advice and n-3 supplementation in newly diagnosed MS patients. *Acta Neurol Scand.* 2000;102(3):143-149.

52. Swank RL, Dugan BB. Effect of low saturated fat diet in early and late cases of multiple sclerosis. *Lancet.* 1990;336(8706):37-39.

53. Bates D. Dietary lipids and multiple sclerosis. *Ups J Med Sci Suppl.* 1990;48:173-187.

54. Perlmutter D. *BrainRecovery.com.* Naples, Florida: Perlmutter Health Center; 2000.

55. Shukla VK, Jensen GE, Clausen J. Erythrocyte glutathione perioxidase deficiency in multiple sclerosis. *Acta Neurol Scand.* 1977;56(6):542-550.

56. Calabrese V, Raffaele R, Cosentino E, Rizza V. Changes in cerebrospinal fluid levels of malondialdehyde and glutathione reductase activity in multiple sclerosis. *Int J Clin Pharmacol Res.* 1994;14(4):119-123.

57. Payne A. Nutrition and diet in the clinical management of multiple sclerosis. *J Hum Nutr Diet.* 2001;14(5):349-357.

58. Besler HT, Comoglu S. Lipoprotein oxidation, plasma total antioxidant capacity and homocysteine level in patients with multiple sclerosis. *Nutr Neurosci.* 2003;6(3):189-196.

59. Clausen J, Jensen GE, Nielsen SA. Selenium in chronic neurologic diseases. Multiple sclerosis and Batten's disease. *Biol Trace Elem Res.* 1988;15:179-203.

60. Mai J, Sorensen PS, Hansen JC. High dose antioxidant supplementation to MS patients. Effects on glutathione peroxidase, clinical safety, and absorption of selenium. *Biol Trace Elem Res.* 1990;24(2):109-117.

61. Rieckmann P, Albrecht M, Kitze B, et al. Tumor necrosis factor-alpha messenger RNA expression in patients with relapsing-remitting multiple sclerosis is associated with disease activity. *Ann Neurol.* 1995;37(1):82-88.

62. Lehmann D, Karussis D, Misrachi-Koll R, Shezen E, Ovadia H, Abramsky O. Oral administration of the oxidant-scavenger N-acetyl-L-cysteine inhibits acute experimental autoimmune encephalomyelitis. *J Neuroimmunol.* 1994;50(1):35-42.

63. Weiss A, Goldman S, Ben Shlomo I, Eyali V, Leibovitz S, Shalev E. Mechanisms of matrix metalloproteinase-9 and matrix metalloproteinase-2 inhibition by N-acetylcysteine in the human term decidua and fetal membranes. *Am J Obstet Gynecol.*

2003;189(6):1758-1763.

64. Galis ZS, Asanuma K, Godin D, Meng X. N-acetyl-cysteine decreases the matrix-degrading capacity of macrophage-derived foam cells: new target for antioxidant therapy? *Circulation.* 1998;97(24):2445-2453.

65. Ramanathan M, Weinstock-Guttman B, Nguyen LT, et al. In vivo gene expression revealed by cDNA arrays: the pattern in relapsing-remitting multiple sclerosis patients compared with normal subjects. *J Neuroimmunol.* 2001;116(2):213-219.

66. Kouwenhoven M, Ozenci V, Gomes A, et al. Multiple sclerosis: elevated expression of matrix metalloproteinases in blood monocytes. *J Autoimmun.* 2001;16(4):463-470.

67. Monastra G, Cross AH, Bruni A, Raine CS. Phosphatidylserine, a putative inhibitor of tumor necrosis factor, prevents autoimmune demyelination. *Neurology.* 1993;43(1):153-163.

68. Reynolds EH. Multiple sclerosis and vitamin B12 metabolism. *J Neuroimmunol.* 1992;40(2-3):225-230.

69. Sandyk R, Awerbuch GI. Vitamin B12 and its relationship to age of onset of multiple sclerosis. *Int J Neurosci.* 1993;71(1-4):93-99.

70. Goodkin DE, Jacobsen DW, Galvez N, Daughtry M, Secic M, Green R. Serum cobalamin deficiency is uncommon in multiple sclerosis. *Arch Neurol.* 1994;51(11):1110-1114.

71. Frequin ST, Wevers RA, Braam M, Barkhof F, Hommes OR. Decreased vitamin B12 and folate levels in cerebrospinal fluid and serum of multiple sclerosis patients after high-dose intravenous methylprednisolone. *J Neurol.* 1993;240(5):305-308.

72. Kira J, Tobimatsu S, Goto I. Vitamin B12 metabolism and massive-dose methyl vitamin B12 therapy in Japanese patients with multiple sclerosis. *Intern Med.* 1994;33(2):82-86.

73. Nieves J, Cosman F, Herbert J, Shen V, Lindsay R. High prevalence of vitamin D deficiency and reduced bone mass in multiple sclerosis. *Neurology.* 1994;44(9):1687-1692.

74. Hayes CE. Vitamin D: a natural inhibitor of multiple sclerosis. *Proc Nutr Soc.* 2000;59(4):531-535.

75. Hayes CE, Cantorna MT, DeLuca HF. Vitamin D and multiple sclerosis. *Proc Soc Exp Biol Med.* 1997;216(1):21-27.

76. Mattner F, Smiroldo S, Galbiati F, et al. Inhibition of Th1 development and treatment of chronic-relapsing experimental allergic encephalomyelitis by a non-hypercalcemic analogue of 1,25-dihydroxyvitamin D(3). *Eur J Immunol.* 2000;30(2):498-508.

77. Nashold FE, Miller DJ, Hayes CE. 1,25-dihydroxyvitamin D3 treatment decreases macrophage accumulation in the CNS of mice with experimental autoimmune encephalomyelitis. *J Neuroimmunol.* 2000;103(2):171-179.

78. Vieth R. Vitamin D supplementation, 25-hydroxyvitamin D concentrations, and safety. *Am J Clin Nutr.* 1999;69(5):842-856.

79. Sandyk R, Awerbuch GI. Nocturnal plasma melatonin and alpha-melanocyte stimulating hormone levels during exacerbation of multiple sclerosis. *Int J Neurosci.* 1992;67(1-4):173-186.

80. Sandyk R. Multiple sclerosis: the role of puberty and the pineal gland in its pathogenesis. *Int J Neurosci.* 1993;68(3-4):209-225.

81. Gupta JK, Ingegno AP, Cook AW, Pertschuk LP. Multiple sclerosis and malabsorption. *Am J Gastroenterol.* 1977;68(6):560-565.

82. Lange LS, Shiner M. Small-bowel abnormalities in multiple sclerosis. *Lancet.* 1976;2(7999):1319-1322.

83. See note 54 above.

84. Sriram S, Stratton CW, Yao S, et al. Chlamydia pneumoniae infection of the central nervous system in multiple sclerosis. *Ann Neurol.* 1999;46(1):6-14.

85. Layh-Schmitt G, Bendl C, Hildt U, et al. Evidence for infection with Chlamydia pneumoniae in a subgroup of patients with multiple sclerosis. *Ann Neurol.* 2000;47(5):652-655.

86. Ke Z, Lu F, Roblin P, Boman J, Hammerschlag MR, Kalman B. Lack of detectable Chlamydia pneumoniae in brain lesions of patients with multiple sclerosis. *Ann Neurol.* 2000;48(3):400.

87. Hauser SL, Doolittle TH, Lopez-Bresnahan M, et al. An antispasticity effect of threonine in multiple sclerosis. *Arch Neurol.* 1992;49(9):923-926.

88. Yasui M, Yase Y, Ando K, Adachi K, Mukoyama M, Ohsugi K. Magnesium concentration in brains from multiple sclerosis patients. *Acta Neurol Scand.* 1990;81(3):197-200.

89. Fujimori H, Yasuda M, Pan-Hou H. Enhancement of cellular adenosine triphosphate levels in PC12 cells by extracellular adenosine. *Biol Pharm Bull.* 2002;25(3):307-311.

90. Toncev G, Milicic B, Toncev S, Samardzic G. Serum uric acid levels in multiple sclerosis patients correlate with activity of disease and blood-brain barrier dysfunction. *Eur J Neurol.* 2002;9(3):221-226.

91. Drulovic J, Dujmovic I, Stojsavljevic N, et al. Uric acid levels in sera from patients with multiple sclerosis. *J Neurol.* 2001;248(2):121-126.

92. Spitsin S, Hooper DC, Leist T, Streletz LJ, Mikheeva T, Koprowskil H. Inactivation of peroxynitrite in multiple sclerosis patients after oral administration of inosine may suggest possible approaches to therapy of the disease. *Mult Scler.* 2001;7(5):313-319.

93. Marton A, Pacher P, Murthy KG, Nemeth ZH, Hasko G, Szabo C. Anti-inflammatory effects of inosine in human monocytes, neutrophils and epithelial cells in vitro. *Int J Mol Med.* 2001;8(6):617-621.

94. Chen P, Goldberg DE, Kolb B, Lanser M, Benowitz LI. Inosine induces axonal rewiring and improves behavioral outcome after stroke. *Proc Natl Acad Sci U S A.* 2002;99(13):9031-9036.

95. Farmer S. Personal communication.

96. Scott GS, Spitsin SV, Kean RB, Mikheeva T, Koprowski H, Hooper DC. Therapeutic intervention in experimental allergic encephalomyelitis by administration of uric acid precursors. *Proc Natl Acad Sci U S A.* 2002;99(25):16303-16308. Epub 12002 Nov 16325.

97. See note 92 above.

98. Constantinescu CS, Freitag P, Kappos L. Increase in serum levels of uric acid, an endogenous antioxidant, under treatment with glatiramer acetate for multiple sclerosis. *Mult Scler.* 2000;6(6):378-381.

99. Sarchielli P, Greco L, Floridi A, Gallai V. Excitatory amino acids and multiple sclerosis: evidence from cerebrospinal fluid. *Arch Neurol.* 2003;60(8):1082-1088.

100. Pitt D, Nagelmeier IE, Wilson HC, Raine CS. Glutamate uptake by oligodendrocytes: Implications for excitotoxicity in multiple sclerosis. *Neurology.* 2003;61(8):1113-1120.

101. Werner P, Pitt D, Raine CS. Multiple sclerosis: altered glutamate homeostasis in lesions correlates with oligodendrocyte and axonal damage. *Ann Neurol.* 2001;50(2):169-180.

102. Matute C, Domercq M, Fogarty DJ, Pascual de Zulueta M, Sanchez-Gomez MV. On how altered glutamate homeostasis may contribute to demyelinating diseases of the CNS. *Adv Exp Med Biol.* 1999;468:97-107.

103. Rosin C, Bates TE, Skaper SD. Excitatory amino acid induced oligodendrocyte cell death in vitro: receptor-dependent and -independent mechanisms. *J Neurochem.* 2004;90(5):1173-1185.

104. Matute C, Alberdi E, Domercq M, Perez-Cerda F, Perez-Samartin A, Sanchez-Gomez MV. The link between excitotoxic oligodendroglial death and demyelinating diseases. *Trends Neurosci.* 2001;24(4):224-230.

105. Werner P, Pitt D, Raine CS. Glutamate excitotoxicity–a mechanism for axonal damage and oligodendrocyte death in Multiple Sclerosis? *J Neural Transm Suppl.* 2000(60):375-385.

106. Pitt D, Werner P, Raine CS. Glutamate excitotoxicity in a model of multiple sclerosis. *Nat Med.* 2000;6(1):67-70.

107. See Note 101 above.

108. Rieckmann P, Maurer M. Anti-inflammatory strategies to prevent axonal injury in multiple sclerosis. *Curr Opin Neurol.* 2002;15(3):361-370.

109. Kidd PM. Multiple sclerosis, an autoimmune inflammatory disease: prospects for its integrative management. *Altern Med Rev.* 2001;6(6):540-566.

110. Owens T. The enigma of multiple sclerosis: inflammation and neurodegeneration cause heterogeneous dysfunction and damage. *Curr Opin Neurol.* 2003;16(3):259-265.

111. Rose JW, Hill KE, Watt HE, Carlson NG. Inflammatory cell expression of cyclooxygenase-2 in the multiple sclerosis lesion. *J Neuroimmunol.* 2004;149(1-2):40-49.

112. See note 101 above.

113. See note 102 above.

114. Chan MM. Inhibition of tumor necrosis factor by curcumin, a phytochemical. *Biochem Pharmacol.* 1995;49(11):1551-1556.

115. Matzner Y, Sallon S. The effect of Padma-28, a traditional Tibetan herbal preparation, on human neutrophil function. *J Clin Lab Immunol.* 1995;46(1):13-23.

116. Badmaev V, Kozlowski PB, Schuller-Levis GB, Wisniewski HM. The therapeutic effect of an herbal formula Badmaev 28 (padma 28) on experimental allergic encephalomyelitis (EAE) in SJL/J mice. *Phytother Res.* 1999;13(3):218-221.

117. Brzosko. Padma 28, a new supplement for patients with HBsAg positive or negative chronic aggressive hepatitis. *Hepatology, Rapid Literature Review 8.* 1982;Memo-H-1971.

118. Korwin-Piotrowska T. Experience of Padma 28 in Multiple Sclerosis. *Phytotherapy Research.* 1991;6:133-136.

119. Brochet B, Guinot P, Orgogozo JM, Confavreux C, Rumbach L, Lavergne V. Double blind placebo controlled multicentre study of ginkgolide B in treatment of acute exacerbations of multiple sclerosis. The Ginkgolide Study Group in multiple sclerosis. *J Neurol Neurosurg Psychiatry.* 1995;58(3):360-362.

120. Petajan JH, Gappmaier E, White AT, Spencer MK, Mino L, Hicks RW. Impact of aerobic training on fitness and quality of life in multiple sclerosis. *Ann Neurol.* 1996;39(4):432-441.

121. Spencer JW, Jacobs JJ. *Complementary/Alternative Medicine, An Evidence Based Approach.* Philadelphia, Pennsylvania: Mosby; 1999.

122. Maguire BL. The effects of imagery on attitudes and moods in multiple sclerosis patients. *Altern Ther Health Med.* 1996;2(5):75-79.

123. Rodgers D, Khoo K, MacEachen M, Oven M, Beatty WW. Cognitive therapy for multiple sclerosis: a preliminary study. *Altern Ther Health Med.* 1996;2(5):70-74.

124. Lang AE, Lozano AM. Parkinson's disease. First of two parts. *N Engl J Med.* 1998;339(15):1044-1053.

125. Abbott RD, Ross GW, White LR, et al. Environmental, life-style, and physical precursors of clinical Parkinson's disease: recent findings from the Honolulu-Asia Aging Study. *J Neurol.* 2003;250(Suppl 3):III30-39.

126. Hellenbrand W, Boeing H, Robra BP, et al. Diet and Parkinson's disease. II: A possible role for the past intake of specific nutrients. Results from a self-administered food-frequency questionnaire in a case-control study. *Neurology.* 1996;47(3):644-650.

127. Powers KM, Smith-Weller T, Franklin GM, Longstreth WT, Jr., Swanson PD, Checkoway H. Parkinson's disease risks associated with dietary iron, manganese, and other nutrient intakes. *Neurology.* 2003;60(11):1761-1766.

128. Gerlach M, Double KL, Ben-Shachar D, Zecca L, Youdim MB, Riederer P. Neuromelanin and its interaction with iron as a potential risk factor for dopaminergic neurodegeneration underlying Parkinson's disease. *Neurotox Res.* 2003;5(1-2):35-44.

129. Zhang SM, Hernan MA, Chen H, Spiegelman D, Willett WC, Ascherio A. Intakes of vitamins E and C, carotenoids, vitamin supplements, and PD risk. *Neurology.* 2002;59(8):1161-1169.

130. Abbott RA, Cox M, Markus H, Tomkins A. Diet, body size and micronutrient status in Parkinson's disease. *Eur J Clin Nutr.* 1992;46(12):879-884.

131. Gao HM, Liu B, Zhang W, Hong JS. Novel anti-inflammatory therapy for Parkinson's disease. *Trends Pharmacol Sci.* 2003;24(8):395-401.

132. Liu B, Gao HM, Hong JS. Parkinson's disease and exposure to infectious agents and pesticides and the occurrence of brain injuries: role of neuroinflammation. *Environ Health Perspect.* 2003;111(8):1065-1073.

133. Barcia C, Fernandez Barreiro A, Poza M, Herrero MT. Parkinson's disease and inflammatory changes. *Neurotox Res.* 2003;5(6):411-418.

134. Astarloa R, Mena MA, Sanchez V, de la Vega L, de Yebenes JG. Clinical and pharmacokinetic effects of a diet rich in insoluble fiber on Parkinson disease. *Clin Neuropharmacol.* 1992;15(5):375-380.

135. Vilmin ST. Diet Therapy in Parkinson's Disease (Norwegian). *Tidsskr Nor Laegeforen.* 1995;115(10):1244-1247.

136. Berry EM, Growdon JH, Wurtman JJ, Caballero B, Wurtman RJ. A balanced carbohydrate: protein diet in the management of Parkinson's disease. *Neurology.* 1991;41(8):1295-1297.

137. Bandmann O, Vaughan JR, Holmans P, Marsden CD, Wood NW. Detailed genotyping demonstrates association between the slow acetylator genotype for N-acetyltransferase 2 (NAT2) and familial Parkinson's disease. *Mov Disord.* 2000;15(1):30-35.

138. Carmine A, Buervenich S, Sydow O, Anvret M, Olson L. Further evidence for an association of the paraoxonase 1 (PON1) Met-54 allele with Parkinson's disease. *Mov Disord.* 2002;17(4):764-766.

139. Tanner CM. Abnormal liver enzyme-mediated metabolism in Parkinson's disease: a second look. *Neurology.* 1991;41(5 Suppl 2):89-91; discussion 92.

140. Yang MC, McLean AJ, Le Couteur DG. Age-related alteration in hepatic disposition of the neurotoxin 1-methyl-4-phenyl-1,2,3,6-tetrahydropyridine and pesticides. *Pharmacol Toxicol.* 2002;90(4):203-207.

141. See note 125 above.

142. Baldereschi M, Di Carlo A, Vanni P, et al. Lifestyle-related risk factors for Parkinson's disease: a population-based study. *Acta Neurol Scand.* 2003;108(4):239-244.

143. Di Monte DA, Lavasani M, Manning-Bog AB. Environmental factors in Parkinson's disease. *Neurotoxicology.* 2002;23(4-5):487-502.

144. Engel LS, Checkoway H, Keifer MC, et al. Parkinsonism and occupational exposure to pesticides. *Occup Environ Med.* 2001;58(9):582-589.

145. Fall PA, Fredrikson M, Axelson O, Granerus AK. Nutritional and occupational factors influencing the risk of Parkinson's disease: a case-control study in southeastern Sweden. *Mov Disord.* 1999;14(1):28-37.

146. Gorell JM, Johnson CC, Rybicki BA, Peterson EL, Richardson RJ. The risk of Parkinson's disease with exposure to pesticides, farming, well water, and rural living. *Neurology.* 1998;50(5):1346-1350.

147. Petrovitch H, Ross GW, Abbott RD, et al. Plantation work and risk of Parkinson disease in a population-based longitudinal study. *Arch Neurol.* 2002;59(11):1787-1792.

148. Priyadarshi A, Khuder SA, Schaub EA, Shrivastava S. A meta-analysis of Parkinson's disease and exposure to pesticides. *Neurotoxicology.* 2000;21(4):435-440.

149. Ritz B, Yu F. Parkinson's disease mortality and pesticide exposure in California 1984-1994. *Int J Epidemiol.* 2000;29(2):323-329.

150. Semchuk KM, Love EJ, Lee RG. Parkinson's disease and exposure to agricultural work and pesticide chemicals. *Neurology.* 1992;42(7):1328-1335.

151. See Note 149 above.

152. See Note 150 above.

153. Grasbon-Frodl EM, Kosel S, Sprinzl M, von Eitzen U, Mehraein P, Graeber MB. Two novel point mutations of mitochondrial tRNA genes in histologically confirmed Parkinson disease. *Neurogenetics.* 1999;2(2):121-127.

154. Fleming L, Mann JB, Bean J, Briggle T, Sanchez-Ramos JR. Parkinson's disease and brain levels of organochlorine pesticides. *Ann Neurol.* 1994;36(1):100-103.

155. See Note 145 above.

156. Pizzorno JJ, Murray M. *Textbook of Natural Medicine.* 2 ed: Churchill Livingston; 1999.

157. Luglie PF, Filia G, Chessa G, Calaresu G. [In vitro evaluation of mercury leakage from dental amalgam using atomic absorption spectrophotometry]. *Minerva Stomatol.* 1999;48(6):239-245.

158. Ngim CH, Devathasan G. Epidemiologic study on the association between body burden mercury level and idiopathic Parkinson's disease. *Neuroepidemiology.* 1989;8(3):128-141.

159. Seidler A, Hellenbrand W, Robra BP, et al. Possible environmental, occupational, and other etiologic factors for Parkinson's disease: a case-control study in Germany. *Neurology.* 1996;46(5):1275-1284.

160. Gorell JM, Johnson CC, Rybicki BA, et al. Occupational exposures to metals as risk factors for Parkinson's disease. *Neurology.* 1997;48(3):650-658.

161. Zecca L, Tampellini D, Gatti A, et al. The neuromelanin of human substantia nigra and its interaction with metals. *J Neural Transm.* 2002;109(5-6):663-672.

162. Di Monte DA, Tokar I, Langston JW. Impaired glutamate clearance as a consequence of energy failure caused by MPP(+) in astrocytic cultures. *Toxicol Appl Pharmacol.* 1999;158(3):296-302.

163. Fallon J, Matthews RT, Hyman BT, Beal MF. MPP+ produces progressive neuronal degeneration which is mediated by oxidative stress. *Exp Neurol.* 1997;144(1):193-198.

164. Levine SA, Kidd PM. *Antioxidant Adaptation, Its Role in Free Radical Pathology*: Allergy Research Group; 1994.

165. Fahn S, Cohen G. The oxidant stress hypothesis in Parkinson's disease: evidence supporting it. *Ann Neurol.* 1992;32(6):804-812.

166. Faucheux BA, Martin ME, Beaumont C, Hauw JJ, Agid Y, Hirsch EC. Neuromelanin associated redox-active iron is increased in the substantia nigra of patients with Parkinson's disease. *J Neurochem.* 2003;86(5):1142-1148.

167. Fahn S. A pilot trial of high-dose alpha-tocopherol and ascorbate in early Parkinson's disease. *Ann Neurol.* 1992;32(Suppl):S128-132.

168. Baker SK, Tarnopolsky MA. Targeting cellular energy production in neurological disorders. *Expert Opin Investig Drugs.* 2003;12(10):1655-1679.

169. Fitzmaurice PS, Ang L, Guttman M, Rajput AH, Furukawa Y, Kish SJ. Nigral glutathione deficiency is not specific for idiopathic Parkinson's disease. *Mov Disord.* 2003;18(9):969-976.

170. Sechi G, Deledda MG, Bua G, et al. Reduced intravenous glutathione in the treatment of early Parkinson's disease. *Prog Neuropsychopharmacol Biol Psychiatry.* 1996;20(7):1159-1170.

171. Lombard J, Germano C. *The Brain Wellness Plan.* New York: Kensington Books; 1997.

172. Kotler M, Rodriguez C, Sainz RM, Antolin I, Menendez-Pelaez A. Melatonin increases gene expression for antioxidant enzymes in rat brain cortex. *J Pineal Res.* 1998;24(2):83-89.

173. Sheu SY, Lai CH, Chiang HC. Inhibition of xanthine oxidase by purpurogallin and silymarin group. *Anticancer Res.* 1998;18(1A):263-267.

174. Swerdlow RH. Is NADH effective in the treatment of Parkinson's disease? *Drugs Aging.* 1998;13(4):263-268.

175. Birkmayer JG, Vrecko C, Volc D, Birkmayer W. Nicotinamide adenine dinucleotide (NADH)–a new therapeutic approach to Parkinson's disease. Comparison of oral and parenteral application. *Acta Neurol Scand Suppl.* 1993;146:32-35.

176. Mukherjee SK, Klaidman LK, Yasharel R, Adams JD, Jr. Increased brain NAD prevents neuronal apoptosis in vivo. *Eur J Pharmacol.* 1997;330(1):27-34.

177. Bastard J, Truelle JL, Emile J. [Effectiveness of 5 hydroxy-tryptophan in Parkinson's disease]. *Nouv Presse Med.* 1976;5(29):1836-1837.

178. Perlmutter D. Toxicity and Neurodegenerative Disorders. Paper presented at: The Sixth International Symposium on Functional Medicine, 1999.

179. Christian B, McConnaughey K, Bethea E, et al. Chronic aspartame affects T-maze performance, brain cholinergic receptors and Na+,K+-ATPase in rats. *Pharmacol Biochem Behav.* 2004;78(1):121-127.

180. Coulombe RA, Jr., Sharma RP. Neurobiochemical alterations induced by the artificial sweetener aspartame (NutraSweet). *Toxicol Appl Pharmacol.* 1986;83(1):79-85.

181. Eguchi K, Yonezawa M, Mitsui Y, Hiramatsu Y. Developmental changes of glutamate dehydrogenase activity in rat liver mitochondria and its enhancement by branched-chain amino acids. *Biol Neonate.* 1992;62(2-3):83-88.

182. Zhou X, Thompson JR. Regulation of glutamate dehydrogenase by branched-chain amino acids in skeletal muscle from rats and chicks. *Int J Biochem Cell Biol.* 1996;28(7):787-793.

183. Molina JA, Jimenez-Jimenez FJ, Gomez P, et al. Decreased cerebrospinal fluid levels of neutral and basic amino acids in patients with Parkinson's disease. *J Neurol Sci.* 1997;150(2):123-127.

184. Patocka J. Huperzine A–an interesting anticholinesterase compound from the Chinese herbal medicine. *Acta Medica (Hradec Kralove).* 1998;41(4):155-157.

185. Cheng DH, Ren H, Tang XC. Huperzine A, a novel promising acetylcholinesterase inhibitor. *Neuroreport.* 1996;8(1):97-101.

186. Engelborghs S, Marescau B, De Deyn PP. Amino acids and biogenic amines in cerebrospinal fluid of patients with Parkinson's disease. *Neurochem Res.* 2003;28(8):1145-1150.

187. El Idrissi A, Trenkner E. Taurine as a modulator of excitatory and inhibitory neurotransmission. *Neurochem Res.* 2004;29(1):189-197.

188. Belluzzi O, Puopolo M, Benedusi M, Kratskin I. Selective neuroinhibitory effects of taurine in slices of rat main olfactory bulb. *Neuroscience.* 2004;124(4):929-944.

189. El Idrissi A, Trenkner E. Taurine regulates mitochondrial calcium homeostasis. *Adv Exp Med Biol.* 2003;526:527-536.

190. El Idrissi A, Trenkner E. Growth factors and taurine protect against excitotoxicity by stabilizing calcium homeostasis and energy metabolism. *J Neurosci.* 1999;19(21):9459-9468.

191. Blaylock R. *Excitotoxins: the taste that kills.* Santa Fe, New Mexico: Health Press; 1997.

192. Louzada PR, Lima AC, Mendonca-Silva DL, Noel F, De Mello FG, Ferreira ST. Taurine prevents the neurotoxicity of beta-amyloid and glutamate receptor agonists: activation of GABA receptors and possible implications for Alzheimer's disease and other neurological disorders. *Faseb J.* 2004;18(3):511-518.

193. Wallace DC, Brown MD, Lott MT. Mitochondrial DNA variation in human evolution and disease. *Gene.* 1999;238(1):211-230.

194. Mecocci P, MacGarvey U, Kaufman AE, et al. Oxidative damage to mitochondrial DNA shows marked age-dependent increases in human brain. *Ann Neurol.* 1993;34(4):609-616.

195. Parker WD, Jr., Swerdlow RH. Mitochondrial dysfunction in idiopathic Parkinson's disease. *Am J Hum Genet.* 1998;62(4):758-762.

196. Mithofer K, Sandy MS, Smith MT, Di Monte D. Mitochondrial poisons cause depletion of reduced glutathione in isolated hepatocytes. *Arch Biochem Biophys.* 1992;295(1):132-136.

197. Kosel S, Hofhaus G, Maassen A, Vieregge P, Graeber MB. Role of mitochondria in Parkinson disease. *Biol Chem.* 1999;380(7-8):865-870.

198. Przedborski S, Jackson-Lewis V, Fahn S. Antiparkinsonian therapies and brain mitochondrial complex I activity. *Mov Disord.* 1995;10(3):312-317.

199. Shults CW, Haas RH, Beal MF. A possible role of coenzyme Q10 in the etiology and treatment of Parkinson's disease. *Biofactors.* 1999;9(2-4):267-272.

200. Shults CW, Oakes D, Kieburtz K, et al. Effects of coenzyme Q10 in early Parkinson's disease: evidence of slowing of the functional decline. *Arch Neurol.* 2002;59(10):1541-1550.

201. Beal MF. Bioenergetic approaches for neuroprotection in Parkinson's disease. *Ann Neurol.* 2003;53(Suppl 3):S39-47; discussion S47-38.

202. Muller T, Buttner T, Gholipour AF, Kuhn W. Coenzyme Q10 supplementation provides mild symptomatic benefit in patients with Parkinson's disease. *Neurosci Lett.* 2003;341(3):201-204.

203. Beal MF. Mitochondria, oxidative damage, and inflammation in Parkinson's disease. *Ann N Y Acad Sci.* 2003;991:120-131.

204. White HL. Extracts of Ginkgo biloba leaves inhibit monoamine oxidase. *Life Science.* 1996;58(16):1315-1321.

205. Lotharius J, Brundin P. Impaired dopamine storage resulting from alpha-synuclein mutations may contribute to the pathogenesis of Parkinson's disease. *Hum Mol Genet.* 2002;11(20):2395-2407.

206. Lucking CB, Brice A. Alpha-synuclein and Parkinson's disease. *Cell Mol Life Sci.* 2000;57(13-14):1894-1908.

207. Jellinger KA. Recent developments in the pathology of Parkinson's disease. *J Neural Transm Suppl.* 2002;(62):347-376.

208. Vanacore N, Nappo A, Gentile M, et al. Evaluation of risk of Parkinson's disease in a cohort of licensed pesticide users. *Neurol Sci.* 2002;23(Suppl 2):S119-120.

209. Hasimoto M. Role of cytochrome c as a stimulator of alpha-synuclein aggregation in Lewy body disease. *J Biol Chem.* 1999;274(41):28849-28852.

210. See Note 133 above.

211. Czlonkowska A, Kurkowska-Jastrzebska I, Czlonkowski A, Peter D, Stefano GB. Immune processes in the pathogenesis of Parkinson's disease–a potential role for microglia and nitric oxide. *Med Sci Monit.* 2002;8(8):RA165-177.

212. Nagatsu T, Mogi M, Ichinose H, Togari A. Changes in cytokines and neurotrophins in Parkinson's disease. *J Neural Transm Suppl.* 2000(60):277-290.

213. Hirsch EC, Breidert T, Rousselet E, Hunot S, Hartmann A, Michel PP. The role of glial reaction and inflammation in Parkinson's disease. *Ann N Y Acad Sci.* 2003;991:214-228.

214. Jara-Prado A, Ortega-Vazquez A, Martinez-Ruano L, Rios C, Santamaria A. Homocysteine-induced brain lipid peroxidation: effects of NMDA receptor blockade, antioxidant treatment, and nitric oxide synthase inhibition. *Neurotox Res.* 2003;5(4):237-243.

215. Rose JW, Hill KE, Watt HE, Carlson NG. Inflammatory cell expression of cyclooxygenase-2 in the multiple sclerosis lesion. *J Neuroimmunol.* 2004;149(1-2):40-49.

216. Shi Q, Savage JE, Hufeisen SJ, et al. L-homocysteine sulfinic acid and other acidic homocysteine derivatives are potent and selective metabotropic glutamate receptor agonists. *J Pharmacol Exp Ther.* 2003;305(1):131-142.

217. Zhang R, Ma J, Xia M, Zhu H, Ling W. Mild hyperhomocysteinemia induced by feeding rats diets rich in methionine or deficient in folate promotes early atherosclerotic inflammatory processes. *J Nutr.* 2004;134(4):825-830.

218. See Note 215 above.

219. Klegeris A, McGeer PL. Cyclooxygenase and 5-lipoxygenase inhibitors protect against mononuclear phagocyte neurotoxicity. *Neurobiol Aging.* 2002;23(5):787-794.

220. LaValle JB. *The Cox-2 Connection.* Rochester, Vermont: Healing Arts Press; 2001.

221. Safayhi H, Boden SE, Schweizer S, Ammon HP. Concentration-dependent potentiating and inhibitory effects of Boswellia extracts on 5-lipoxygenase product formation in stimulated PMNL. *Planta Med.* 2000;66(2):110-113.

222. Resch M, Heilmann J, Steigel A, Bauer R. Further phenols and polyacetylenes from the rhizomes of Atractylodes lancea and their anti-inflammatory activity. *Planta Med.* 2001;67(5):437-442.

223. Hong J, Bose M, Ju J, et al. Modulation of arachidonic acid metabolism by curcumin and related {beta}-diketone derivatives: effects on cytosolic phospholipase A2, cyclooxygenases, and 5-lipoxygenase. *Carcinogenesis.* 2004;8:8.

224. Gupta B, Ghosh B. Curcuma longa inhibits TNF-alpha induced expression of adhesion molecules on human umbilical vein endothelial cells. *Int J Immunopharmacol.* 1999;21(11):745-757.

225. Chun KS, Keum YS, Han SS, Song YS, Kim SH, Surh YJ. Curcumin inhibits phorbol ester-induced expression of cyclooxygenase-2 in mouse skin through suppression of extracellular signal-regulated kinase activity and NF-kappaB activation. *Carcinogenesis.* 2003;24(9):1515-1524. Epub 2003 Jul 1514.

226. Aggarwal BB, Takada Y, Shishodia S, et al. Nuclear transcription factor NF-kappa B: role in biology and medicine. *Indian J Exp Biol.* 2004;42(4):341-353.

227. Janssen-Heininger YM, Poynter ME, Baeuerle PA. Recent advances towards understanding redox mechanisms in the activation of nuclear factor kappaB. *Free Radic Biol Med.* 2000;28(9):1317-1327.

228. Pischon T, Hankinson SE, Hotamisligil GS, Rifai N, Willett WC, Rimm EB. Habitual dietary intake of n-3 and n-6 fatty acids in relation to inflammatory markers among US men and women. *Circulation.* 2003;108(2):155-160. Epub 2003 Jun 2023.

229. Dhindsa S, Tripathy D, Mohanty P, et al. Differential effects of glucose and alcohol on reactive oxygen species generation and intranuclear nuclear factor-kappaB in mononuclear cells. *Metabolism.* 2004;53(3):330-334.

230. Keller JN, Hanni KB, Markesbery WR. Possible involvement of proteasome inhibition in aging: implications for oxidative stress. *Mech Ageing Dev.* 2000;113(1):61-70.

231. Zeng BY, Medhurst AD, Jackson M, Rose S, Jenner P. Proteasomal activity in brain differs between species and brain regions and changes with age. *Mech Ageing Dev.* 2005;126(6-7):760-766. Epub 2005 Mar 2005.

232. Sullivan PG, Dragicevic NB, Deng JH, et al. Proteasome inhibition alters neural mitochondrial homeostasis and mitochondria turnover. *J Biol Chem.* 2004;279(20):20699-20707. Epub 22004 Jan 20622.

233. Keck S, Nitsch R, Grune T, Ullrich O. Proteasome inhibition by paired helical filament-tau in brains of patients with Alzheimer's disease. *J Neurochem.* Apr 2003;85(1):115-122.

234. McNaught KS, Jenner P. Proteasomal function is impaired in substantia nigra in Parkinson's disease. *Neurosci Lett.* 2001;297(3):191-194.

235. Snyder H, Wolozin B. Pathological proteins in Parkinson's disease: focus on the proteasome. *J Mol Neurosci.* 2004;24(3):425-442.

236. Wojcik C, Di Napoli M. Ubiquitin-proteasome system and proteasome inhibition: new strategies in stroke therapy. *Stroke.* 2004;35(6):1506-1518. Epub 2004 Apr 1529.

237. Hosseini H, Andre P, Lefevre N, et al. Protection against experimental autoimmune encephalomyelitis by a proteasome modulator. *J Neuroimmunol.* 2001;118(2):233-244.

238. Olas B, Wachowicz B. Resveratrol and vitamin C as antioxidants in blood platelets. *Thromb Res.* 2002;106(2):143-148.

239. Granados-Soto V. Pleiotropic effects of resveratrol. *Drug News Perspect.* 2003;16(5):299-307.

240. Cal C, Garban H, Jazirehi A, Yeh C, Mizutani Y, Bonavida B. Resveratrol and cancer: chemoprevention, apoptosis, and chemo-immunosensitizing activities. *Curr Med Chem Anticancer Agents.* 2003;3(2):77-93.

241. Pervaiz S. Chemotherapeutic potential of the chemopreventive phytoalexin resveratrol. *Drug Resist Updat.* 2004;7(6):333-344. Epub 2004 Dec 2019.

242. Zaslaver M, Offer S, Kerem Z, et al. Natural compounds derived from foods modulate nitric oxide production and oxidative status in epithelial lung cells. *J Agric Food Chem.* 2005;53(26):9934-9939.

243. Rogina B, Helfand SL. Sir2 mediates longevity in the fly through a pathway related to calorie restriction. *Proc Natl Acad Sci U S A.* 2004;101(45):15998-16003. Epub 12004 Nov 15991.

244. Guarente L. Calorie restriction and SIR2 genes–towards a mechanism. *Mech Ageing Dev.* 2005;126(9):923-928.

245. Howitz KT, Bitterman KJ, Cohen HY, et al. Small molecule activators of sirtuins extend Saccharomyces cerevisiae lifespan. *Nature.* 2003;425(6954):191-196. Epub 2003 Aug 2024.

246. Marambaud P, Zhao H, Davies P. Resveratrol promotes clearance of Alzheimer's disease amyloid-beta peptides. *J Biol Chem.* 2005;280(45):37377-37382. Epub 32005 Sep 37314.

247. Hart AM, Terenghi G, Kellerth JO, Wiberg M. Sensory neuroprotection, mitochondrial preservation, and therapeutic potential of n-acetyl-cysteine after nerve injury. *Neuroscience.* 2004;125(1):91-101.

248. Ornaghi F, Ferrini S, Prati M, Giavini E. The protective effects of N-acetyl-L-cysteine against methyl mercury embryotoxicity in mice. *Fundam Appl Toxicol.* 1993;20(4):437-445.

249. Kasparova J, Dolezal V. [beta-Amyloid, cholinergic neurons and Alzheimer's disease]. *Cesk Fysiol.* 2002;51(2):82-94.

250. Mark RJ, Blanc EM, Mattson MP. Amyloid beta-peptide and oxidative cellular injury in Alzheimer's disease. *Mol Neurobiol.* 1996;12(3):211-224.

251. Lukiw WJ, Bazan NG. Neuroinflammatory signaling upregulation in Alzheimer's disease. *Neurochem Res.* 2000;25(9-10):1173-1184.

252. Pei JJ, Gong CX, Iqbal K, et al. Subcellular distribution of protein phosphatases and abnormally phosphorylated tau in the temporal cortex from Alzheimer's disease and control brains. *J Neural Transm.* 1998;105(1):69-83.

253. Cedazo-Minguez A, Cowburn RF. Apolipoprotein E: a major piece in the Alzheimer's disease puzzle. *J Cell Mol Med.* 2001;5(3):254-266.

254. Studer R, Baysang G, Brack C. N-Acetyl-L-Cystein downregulates beta-amyloid precursor protein gene transcription in human neuroblastoma cells. *Biogerontology.* 2001;2(1):55-60.

255. Adair JC, Knoefel JE, Morgan N. Controlled trial of N-acetylcysteine for patients with probable Alzheimer's disease. *Neurology.* 2001;57(8):1515-1517.

256. Mackenzie IR, Munoz DG. Nonsteroidal anti-inflammatory drug use and Alzheimer-type pathology in aging. *Neurology.* 1998;50(4):986-990.

257. Thomas T, Nadackal TG, Thomas K. Aspirin and non-steroidal anti-inflammatory drugs inhibit amyloid-beta aggregation. *Neuroreport.* 2001;12(15):3263-3267.

258. Lim GP, Chu T, Yang F, Beech W, Frautschy SA, Cole GM. The curry spice curcumin reduces oxidative damage and amyloid pathology in an Alzheimer transgenic mouse. *J Neurosci.* 2001;21(21):8370-8377.

259. Ono K, Hasegawa K, Naiki H, Yamada M. Curcumin has potent anti-amyloidogenic effects for Alzheimer's beta-amyloid fibrils in vitro. *J Neurosci Res.* 2004;75(6):742-750.

260. Yatin SM, Varadarajan S, Butterfield DA. Vitamin E Prevents Alzheimer's Amyloid-beta-peptide (1-42)-Induced Neuronal Protein Oxidation and Reactive Oxygen Species Production. *J Alzheimers Dis.* 2000;2(2):123-131.

261. Tabet N, Mantle D, Walker Z, Orrell M. Endogenous antioxidant activities in relation to concurrent vitamins A, C, and E intake in dementia. *Int Psychogeriatr.* 2002;14(1):7-15.

262. Grundman M. Vitamin E and Alzheimer disease: the basis for additional clinical trials. *Am J Clin Nutr.* 2000;71(2):630S-636S.

263. Sano M, Ernesto C, Thomas RG, et al. A controlled trial of selegiline, alpha-tocopherol, or both as treatment for Alzheimer's disease. The Alzheimer's Disease Cooperative Study. *N Engl J Med.* 1997;336(17):1216-1222.

264. Kontush A, Mann U, Arlt S, et al. Influence of vitamin E and C supplementation on lipoprotein oxidation in patients with Alzheimer's disease. *Free Radic Biol Med.* 2001;31(3):345-354.

265. Peng QL, Buz'Zard AR, Lau BH. Pycnogenol protects neurons from amyloid-beta peptide-induced apoptosis. *Brain Res Mol Brain Res.* 2002;104(1):55-65.

266. TherapeuticResearchFaculty. *Natural Medicines: Comprehensive Database.* Stockton: Therapeutic Research Center; 2002.

267. Peng Q, Buz'Zard AR, Lau BH. Neuroprotective effect of garlic compounds in amyloid-beta peptide-induced apoptosis in vitro. *Med Sci Monit.* 2002;8(8):BR328-337.

268. Bastianetto S, Ramassamy C, Dore S, Christen Y, Poirier J, Quirion R. The Ginkgo biloba extract (EGb 761) protects hippocampal neurons against cell death induced by beta-amyloid. *Eur J Neurosci.* 2000;12(6):1882-1890.

269. Schindowski K, Leutner S, Kressmann S, Eckert A, Muller WE. Age-related increase of oxidative stress-induced apoptosis in mice prevention by Ginkgo biloba extract (EGb761). *J Neural Transm.* 2001;108(8-9):969-978.

270. Luo Y, Smith JV, Paramasivam V, et al. Inhibition of amyloid-beta aggregation and caspase-3 activation by the Ginkgo biloba extract EGb761. *Proc Natl Acad Sci U S A.* 2002;99(19):12197-12202. Epub 12002 Sep 12194.

271. Le Bars PL, Katz MM, Berman N, Itil TM, Freedman AM, Schatzberg AF. A placebo-controlled, double-blind, randomized trial of an extract of Ginkgo biloba for dementia. North American EGb Study Group. *Jama.* 1997;278(16):1327-1332.

272. Le Bars PL, Kieser M, Itil KZ. A 26-week analysis of a double-blind, placebo-controlled trial of the ginkgo biloba extract EGb 761 in dementia. *Dement Geriatr Cogn Disord.* 2000;11(4):230-237.

273. Le Bars PL, Velasco FM, Ferguson JM, Dessain EC, Kieser M, Hoerr R. Influence of the severity of cognitive impairment on the effect of the Gnkgo biloba extract EGb 761 in Alzheimer's disease. *Neuropsychobiology.* 2002;45(1):19-26.

274. Wettstein A. Cholinesterase inhibitors and Gingko extracts–are they comparable in the treatment of dementia? Comparison of published placebo-controlled efficacy studies of at least six months' duration. *Phytomedicine.* 2000;6(6):393-401.

275. Shen YX, Xu SY, Wei W, et al. The protective effects of melatonin from oxidative damage induced by amyloid-beta-peptide 25-35 in middle-aged rats. *J Pineal Res.* 2002;32(2):85-89.

276. Daniels WM, van Rensburg SJ, van Zyl JM, Taljaard JJ. Melatonin prevents beta-amyloid-induced lipid peroxidation. *J Pineal Res.* 1998;24(2):78-82.

277. Lahiri DK. Melatonin affects the metabolism of the beta-amyloid precursor protein in different cell types. *J Pineal Res.* 1999;26(3):137-146.

278. See note 266 above.

279. Clarke R, Smith AD, Jobst KA, Refsum H, Sutton L, Ueland PM. Folate, vitamin B12, and serum total homocysteine levels in confirmed Alzheimer disease. *Arch Neurol.* 1998;55(11):1449-1455.

280. Miller JW. Homocysteine and Alzheimer's disease. *Nutr Rev.* 1999;57(4):126-129.

281. Vafai SB, Stock JB. Protein phosphatase 2A methylation: a link between elevated plasma homocysteine and Alzheimer's Disease. *FEBS Lett.* 2002;518(1-3):1-4.

282. Hogervorst E, Ribeiro HM, Molyneux A, Budge M, Smith AD. Plasma homocysteine levels, cerebrovascular risk factors, and cerebral white matter changes (leukoaraiosis) in patients with Alzheimer disease. *Arch Neurol.* 2002;59(5):787-793.

283. Miller JW, Green R, Mungas DM, Reed BR, Jagust WJ. Homocysteine, vitamin B6, and vascular disease in AD patients. *Neurology.* 2002;58(10):1471-1475.

284. Nilsson K, Gustafson L, Hultberg B. Relation between plasma homocysteine and Alzheimer's disease. *Dement Geriatr Cogn Disord.* 2002;14(1):7-12.

285. See Note 266 above.

286. Delwaide PJ, Gyselynck-Mambourg AM, Hurlet A, Ylieff M. Double-blind randomized controlled study of phosphatidylserine in senile demented patients. *Acta Neurol Scand.* 1986;73(2):136-140.

287. Engel RR, Satzger W, Gunther W, et al. Double-blind cross-over study of phosphatidylserine vs. placebo in patients with early dementia of the Alzheimer type. *Eur Neuropsychopharmacol.* 1992;2(2):149-155.

288. Crook T, Petrie W, Wells C, Massari DC. Effects of phosphatidylserine in Alzheimer's disease. *Psychopharmacol Bull.* 1992;28(1):61-66.

289. Schreiber S, Kampf-Sherf O, Gorfine M, Kelly D, Oppenheim Y, Lerer B. An open trial of plant-source derived phosphatydilserine for treatment of age-related cognitive decline. *Isr J Psychiatry Relat Sci.* 2000;37(4):302-307.

290. See Note 266 above.

291. Virmani MA, Caso V, Spadoni A, Rossi S, Russo F, Gaetani F. The action of acetyl-L-carnitine on the neurotoxicity evoked by amyloid fragments and peroxide on primary rat cortical neurones. *Ann N Y Acad Sci.* 2001;939:162-178.

292. Montgomery SA, Thal LJ, Amrein R. Meta-analysis of double blind randomized controlled clinical trials of acetyl-L-carnitine versus placebo in the treatment of mild cognitive impairment and mild Alzheimer's disease. *Int Clin Psychopharmacol.* 2003;18(2):61-71.

293. Spagnoli A, Lucca U, Menasce G, et al. Long-term acetyl-L-carnitine treatment in Alzheimer's disease. *Neurology.* 1991;41(11):1726-1732.

294. Thal LJ, Carta A, Clarke WR, et al. A 1-year multicenter placebo-controlled study of acetyl-L-carnitine in patients with Alzheimer's disease. *Neurology.* 1996;47(3):705-711.

295. Thal LJ, Calvani M, Amato A, Carta A. A 1-year controlled trial of acetyl-l-carnitine in early-onset AD. *Neurology.* 2000;55(6):805-810.

296. See Note 266 above.

297. Xiao XQ, Zhang HY, Tang XC. Huperzine A attenuates amyloid beta-peptide fragment 25-35-induced apoptosis in rat cortical neurons via inhibiting reactive oxygen species formation and caspase-3 activation. *J Neurosci Res.* 2002;67(1):30-36.

298. Gordon RK, Nigam SV, Weitz JA, Dave JR, Doctor BP, Ved HS. The NMDA receptor ion channel: a site for binding of Huperzine A. *J Appl Toxicol.* 2001;21(Suppl 1):S47-51.

299. Liang YQ, Tang XC. Comparative effects of huperzine A, donepezil and rivastigmine on cortical acetylcholine level and acetylcholinesterase activity in rats. *Neurosci Lett.* 2004;361(1-3):56-59.

300. Zhao Q, Tang XC. Effects of huperzine A on acetylcholinesterase isoforms in vitro: comparison with tacrine, donepezil, rivastigmine and physostigmine. *Eur J Pharmacol.* 2002;455(2-3):101-107.

301. Alcala Mdel M, Vivas NM, Hospital S, Camps P, Munoz-Torrero D, Badia A. Characterisation of the anticholinesterase activity of two new tacrine-huperzine A hybrids. *Neuropharmacology.* 2003;44(6):749-755.

302. Camps P, Munoz-Torrero D. Tacrine-huperzine A hybrids (huprines): a new class of highly potent and selective acetylcholinesterase inhibitors of interest for the treatment of Alzheimer's disease. *Mini Rev Med Chem.* 2001;1(2):163-174.

303. Xu SS, Gao ZX, Weng Z, et al. Efficacy of tablet huperzine-A on memory, cognition, and behavior in Alzheimer's disease. *Zhongguo Yao Li Xue Bao.* 1995;16(5):391-395.

304. Xu SS, Cai ZY, Qu ZW, et al. Huperzine-A in capsules and tablets for treating patients with Alzheimer's disease. *Zhongguo Yao Li Xue Bao.* 1999;20(6):486-490.

305. Jiang H, Luo X, Bai D. Progress in clinical, pharmacological, chemical and structural biological studies of huperzine A: a drug of traditional Chinese medicine origin for the treatment of Alzheimer's disease. *Curr Med Chem.* 2003;10(21):2231-2252.

306. Tully AM, Roche HM, Doyle R, et al. Low serum cholesteryl ester-docosahexaenoic acid levels in Alzheimer's disease: a case-control study. *Br J Nutr.* 2003;89(4):483-489.

307. Hashimoto M, Hossain S, Shimada T, et al. Docosahexaenoic acid provides protection from impairment of learning ability in Alzheimer's disease model rats. *J Neurochem.* 2002;81(5):1084-1091.

308. Flaten TP. Aluminum as a risk factor in Alzheimer's disease, with emphasis on drinking water. *Brain Res Bull.* 2001;55(2):187-196.

309. Yokel RA. The toxicology of aluminum in the brain: a review. *Neurotoxicology.* 2000;21(5):813-828.

310. Campbell A, Bondy SC. Aluminum induced oxidative events and its relation to inflammation: a role for the metal in Alzheimer's disease. *Cell Mol Biol (Noisy-le-grand).* 2000;46(4):721-730.

311. Campbell A. The potential role of aluminum in Alzheimer's disease. *Nephrol Dial Transplant.* 2002;17(Suppl 2):17-20.

312. Pratico D, Uryu K, Sung S, Tang S, Trojanowski JQ, Lee VM. Aluminum modulates brain amyloidosis through oxidative stress in APP transgenic mice. *Faseb J.* 2002;16(9):1138-1140. Epub 2002 May 1121.

313. Perlmutter D. *BrainRecovery.com.* Naples, Florida: Perlmutter Health Center; 2000.

314. Munch G, Schinzel R, Loske C, et al. Alzheimer's disease–synergistic effects of glucose deficit, oxidative stress and advanced glycation endproducts. *J Neural Transm.* 1998;105(4-5):439-461.

315. Dukic-Stefanovic S, Schinzel R, Riederer P, Munch G. AGES in brain ageing: AGE-inhibitors as neuroprotective and anti-dementia drugs? *Biogerontology.* 2001;2(1):19-34.

316. Sobel E, Dunn M, Davanipour Z, Qian Z, Chui HC. Elevated risk of Alzheimer's disease among workers with likely electromagnetic field exposure. *Neurology.* 1996;47(6):1477-1481.

317. Sobel E, Davanipour Z, Sulkava R, et al. Occupations with exposure to electromagnetic fields: a possible risk factor for Alzheimer's disease. *Am J Epidemiol.* 1995;142(5):515-524.

318. Feychting M, Pedersen NL, Svedberg P, Floderus B, Gatz M. Dementia and occupational exposure to magnetic fields. *Scand J Work Environ Health.* 1998;24(1):46-53.

319. Graves AB, Rosner D, Echeverria D, Yost M, Larson EB. Occupational exposure to electromagnetic fields and Alzheimer's disease. *Alzheimer Dis Assoc Disord.* 1999;13(3):165-170.

320. Li CY, Sung FC, Wu SC. Risk of cognitive impairment in relation to elevated exposure to electromagnetic fields. *J Occup Environ Med.* 2002;44(1):66-72.

321. Marino AA, Nilsen E, Frilot C. Nonlinear changes in brain electrical activity due to cell phone radiation. *Bioelectromagnetics.* 2003;24(5):339-346.

322. Sato Y, Asoh T, Oizumi K. High prevalence of vitamin D deficiency and reduced bone mass in elderly women with Alzheimer's disease. *Bone.* 1998;23(6):555-557.

323. Almeida CG, Takahashi RH, Gouras GK. Beta-amyloid accumulation impairs multivesicular body sorting by inhibiting the ubiquitin-proteasome system. *J Neurosci.* Apr 19 2006;26(16):4277-4288.

324. Keck S, Nitsch R, Grune T, Ullrich O. Proteasome inhibition by paired helical filament-tau in brains of patients with Alzheimer's disease. *J Neurochem.* Apr 2003;85(1):115-122.

325. Oh S, Hong H, Hwang E, et al. Amyloid peptide attenuates the proteasome activity in neuronal cells. *Mech Ageing Dev.* 2005;126(12):1292-1299.

326. Marambaud P, Zhao H, Davies P. Resveratrol promotes clearance of Alzheimer's disease amyloid-beta peptides. *J Biol Chem.* 2005;280(45):37377-37382. Epub 32005 Sep 37314.

327. See Note 266 above.

328. Christian B, McConnaughey K, Bethea E, et al. Chronic aspartame affects T-maze performance, brain cholinergic receptors and Na+,K+-ATPase in rats. *Pharmacol Biochem Behav.* 2004;78(1):121-127.

329. Coulombe RA, Jr., Sharma RP. Neurobiochemical alterations induced by the artificial sweetener aspartame (NutraSweet). *Toxicol Appl Pharmacol.* 1986;83(1):79-85.

330. Lesniak W, Kolasinska-Kloch W, Kiec B. [Vascular endothelium–function, disorders and clinical modification probes]. *Folia Med Cracov.* 2001;42(1-2):5-14.

331. Mehta JL, Li DY, Chen HJ, Joseph J, Romeo F. Inhibition of LOX-1 by statins may relate to upregulation of eNOS. *Biochem Biophys Res Commun.* 2001;289(4):857-861.

332. d'Uscio LV, Milstien S, Richardson D, Smith L, Katusic ZS. Long-term vitamin C treatment increases vascular tetrahydrobiopterin levels and nitric oxide synthase activity. *Circ Res.* 2003;92(1):88-95.

333. Amin-Hanjani S, Stagliano NE, Yamada M, Huang PL, Liao JK, Moskowitz MA. Mevastatin, an HMG-CoA reductase inhibitor, reduces stroke damage and upregulates endothelial nitric oxide synthase in mice. *Stroke.* 2001;32(4):980-986.

334. Laufs U, Gertz K, Dirnagl U, Bohm M, Nickenig G, Endres M. Rosuvastatin, a new HMG-CoA reductase inhibitor, upregulates endothelial nitric oxide synthase and protects from ischemic stroke in mice. *Brain Res.* 2002;942(1-2):23-30.

335. Laufs U, Gertz K, Huang P, et al. Atorvastatin upregulates type III nitric oxide synthase in thrombocytes, decreases platelet activation, and protects from cerebral ischemia in normocholesterolemic mice. *Stroke.* 2000;31(10):2442-2449.

336. Mauriello A, Sangiorgi G, Palmieri G, et al. Hyperfibrinogenemia is associated with specific histocytological composition and complications of atherosclerotic carotid plaques in patients affected by transient ischemic attacks. *Circulation.* 2000;101(7):744-750.

337. Rothwell PM, Howard SC, Power DA, et al. Fibrinogen concentration and risk of ischemic stroke and acute coronary events in 5113 patients with transient ischemic attack and minor ischemic stroke. *Stroke.* 2004;35(10):2300-2305. Epub 2004 Sep 2302.

338. Fujita M, Hong K, Ito Y, Fujii R, Kariya K, Nishimuro S. Thrombolytic effect of nattokinase on a chemically induced thrombosis model in rat. *Biol Pharm Bull.* 1995;18(10):1387-1391.

339. Suzuki Y, Kondo K, Ichise H, Tsukamoto Y, Urano T, Umemura K. Dietary supplementation with fermented soybeans suppresses intimal thickening. *Nutrition.* 2003;19(3):261-264.

340. Sumi H, Hamada H, Nakanishi K, Hiratani H. Enhancement of the fibrinolytic activity in plasma by oral administration of nattokinase. *Acta Haematol.* 1990;84(3):139-143.

341. Berg D, Berg LH, Couvaras J, Harrison H. Chronic fatigue syndrome and/or fibromyalgia as a variation of antiphospholipid antibody syndrome: an explanatory model and approach to laboratory diagnosis. *Blood Coagul Fibrinolysis.* 1999;10(7):435-438.

342. Kunt T, Forst T, Wilhelm A, et al. Alpha-lipoic acid reduces expression of vascular cell adhesion molecule-1 and endothelial adhesion of human monocytes after stimulation with advanced glycation end products. *Clin Sci (Lond).* 1999;96(1):75-82.

343. Kagan VE, Serbinova EA, Forte T, Scita G, Packer L. Recycling of vitamin E in human low density lipoproteins. *J Lipid Res.* 1992;33(3):385-397.

344. Bierhaus A, Chevion S, Chevion M, et al. Advanced glycation end product-induced activation of NF-kappaB is suppressed by alpha-lipoic acid in cultured endothelial cells. *Diabetes.* 1997;46(9):1481-1490.

345. Schubert SY, Neeman I, Resnick N. A novel mechanism for the inhibition of NF-kappaB activation in vascular endothelial cells by natural antioxidants. *Faseb J.* 2002;16(14):1931-1933. Epub 2002 Oct 1904.

346. Wiklund O, Fager G, Andersson A, Lundstam U, Masson P, Hultberg B. N-acetylcysteine treatment lowers plasma homocysteine but not serum lipoprotein(a) levels. *Atherosclerosis.* 1996;119(1):99-106.

347. Gavish D, Breslow JL. Lipoprotein(a) reduction by N-acetylcysteine. *Lancet.* 1991;337(8735):203-204.

348. Galis ZS, Asanuma K, Godin D, Meng X. N-acetyl-cysteine decreases the matrix-degrading capacity of macrophage-derived foam cells: new target for antioxidant therapy? *Circulation.* 1998;97(24):2445-2453.

349. Thomas SR, Witting PK, Stocker R. A role for reduced coenzyme Q in atherosclerosis? *Biofactors.* 1999;9(2-4):207-224.

350. Thomas SR, Leichtweis SB, Pettersson K, et al. Dietary cosupplementation with vitamin E and coenzyme Q(10) inhibits atherosclerosis in apolipoprotein E gene knockout mice. *Arterioscler Thromb Vasc Biol.* 2001;21(4):585-593.

351. Singh RB, Neki NS, Kartikey K, et al. Effect of coenzyme Q10 on risk of atherosclerosis in patients with recent myocardial infarction. *Mol Cell Biochem.* 2003;246(1-2):75-82.

352. Witting PK, Pettersson K, Letters J, Stocker R. Anti-atherogenic effect of coenzyme Q10 in apolipoprotein E gene knockout mice. *Free Radic Biol Med.* 2000;29(3-4):295-305.

353. Wang XL, Rainwater DL, Mahaney MC, Stocker R. Cosupplementation with vitamin E and coenzyme Q10 reduces circulating markers of inflammation in baboons. *Am J Clin Nutr.* 2004;80(3):649-655.

354. Brasen JH, Koenig K, Bach H, et al. Comparison of the effects of alpha-tocopherol, ubiquinone-10 and probucol at therapeutic doses on atherosclerosis in WHHL rabbits. *Atherosclerosis.* 2002;163(2):249-259.

355. De Pinieux G, Chariot P, Ammi-Said M, et al. Lipid-lowering drugs and mitochondrial function: effects of HMG-CoA reductase inhibitors on serum ubiquinone and blood lactate/pyruvate ratio. *Br J Clin Pharmacol.* 1996;42(3):333-337.

356. Mortensen SA, Leth A, Agner E, Rohde M. Dose-related decrease of serum coenzyme Q10 during treatment with HMG-CoA reductase inhibitors. *Mol Aspects Med.* 1997;18(Suppl):S137-144.

357. Hosein S. Extra coenzyme Q10 for statin users? *Treatment Update.* 2001;13(2).

358. Passi S, Stancato A, Aleo E, Dmitrieva A, Littarru GP. Statins lower plasma and lymphocyte ubiquinol/ubiquinone without affecting other antioxidants and PUFA. *Biofactors.* 2003;18(1-4):113-124.

359. Mezzetti A, Zuliani G, Romano F, et al. Vitamin E and lipid peroxide plasma levels predict the risk of cardiovascular events in a group of healthy very old people. *J Am Geriatr Soc.* 2001;49(5):533-537.

360. Li D, Saldeen T, Romeo F, Mehta JL. Different isoforms of tocopherols enhance nitric oxide synthase phosphorylation and inhibit human platelet aggregation and lipid peroxidation: implications in therapy with vitamin E. *J Cardiovasc Pharmacol Ther.* 2001;6(2):155-161.

361. Liu M, Wallin R, Wallmon A, Saldeen T. Mixed tocopherols have a stronger inhibitory effect on lipid peroxidation than alpha-tocopherol alone. *J Cardiovasc Pharmacol.* 2002;39(5):714-721.

362. Ascherio A, Rimm EB, Hernan MA, et al. Relation of consumption of vitamin E, vitamin C, and carotenoids to risk for stroke among men in the United States. *Ann Intern Med.* 1999;130(12):963-970.

363. Hodis HN, Mack WJ, LaBree L, et al. Alpha-tocopherol supplementation in healthy individuals reduces low-density lipoprotein oxidation but not atherosclerosis: the Vitamin E Atherosclerosis Prevention Study (VEAPS). *Circulation.* 2002;106(12):1453-1459.

364. Venugopal SK, Devaraj S, Yuhanna I, Shaul P, Jialal I. Demonstration that C-reactive protein decreases eNOS expression and bioactivity in human aortic endothelial cells. *Circulation.* 2002;106(12):1439-1441.

365. Devaraj S, Jialal I. Alpha-tocopherol supplementation decreases serum C-reactive protein and monocyte interleukin-6 levels in normal volunteers and type 2 diabetic patients. *Free Radic Biol Med.* 2000;29(8):790-792.

366. Krajcovicova-Kudlackova M, Ginter E, Blazicek P, Klvanova J. Homocysteine and vitamin C. *Bratisl Lek Listy.* 2002;103(4-5):171-173.

367. Jenner AM, Ruiz JE, Dunster C, Halliwell B, Mann GE, Siow RC. Vitamin C protects against hypochlorous Acid-induced glutathione depletion and DNA base and protein damage in human vascular smooth muscle cells. *Arterioscler Thromb Vasc Biol.* 2002;22(4):574-580.

368. Salonen RM, Nyyssonen K, Kaikkonen J, et al. Six-year effect of combined vitamin C and E supplementation on atherosclerotic progression: the Antioxidant Supplementation in Atherosclerosis Prevention (ASAP) Study. *Circulation.* 2003;107(7):947-953.

369. McCarty MF. Policosanol safely down-regulates HMG-CoA reductase–potential as a component of the Esselstyn regimen. *Med Hypotheses.* 2002;59(3):268-279.

370. Arruzazabala ML, Molina V, Mas R, et al. Antiplatelet effects of policosanol (20 and 40 mg/day) in healthy volunteers and dyslipidaemic patients. *Clin Exp Pharmacol Physiol.* 2002;29(10):891-897.

371. Noa M, Mas R, de la Rosa MC, Magraner J. Effect of policosanol on lipofundin-induced atherosclerotic lesions in rats. *J Pharm Pharmacol.* 1995;47(4):289-291.

372. Arruzazabala ML, Noa M, Menendez R, et al. Protective effect of policosanol on atherosclerotic lesions in rabbits with exogenous hypercholesterolemia. *Braz J Med Biol Res.* 2000;33(7):835-840.

373. Castano G, Mas R, Arruzazabala ML, et al. Effects of policosanol and pravastatin on lipid profile, platelet aggregation and endothelemia in older hypercholesterolemic patients. *Int J Clin Pharmacol Res.* 1999;19(4):105-116.

374. Crespo N, Illnait J, Mas R, Fernandez L, Fernandez J, Castano G. Comparative study of the efficacy and tolerability of policosanol and lovastatin in patients with hypercholesterolemia and noninsulin dependent diabetes mellitus. *Int J Clin Pharmacol Res.* 1999;19(4):117-127.

375. Castano G, Mas R, Fernandez JC, Fernandez L, Illnait J, Lopez E. Effects of policosanol on older patients with hypertension and type II hypercholesterolaemia. *Drugs R D.* 2002;3(3):159-172.

376. Ma J, Li Y, Ye Q, et al. Constituents of red yeast rice, a traditional Chinese food and medicine. *J Agric Food Chem.* 2000;48(11):5220-5225.

377. Man RY, Lynn EG, Cheung F, Tsang PS, O K. Cholestin inhibits cholesterol synthesis and secretion in hepatic cells (HepG2). *Mol Cell Biochem.* 2002;233(1-2):153-158.

378. Heber D, Yip I, Ashley JM, Elashoff DA, Elashoff RM, Go VL. Cholesterol-lowering effects of a proprietary Chinese red-yeast-rice dietary supplement. *Am J Clin Nutr.* 1999;69(2):231-236.

379. Oin S, Zhang W, Oi P. Elderly patients with primary hyperlipidemia benefited from treatment with a Monascus purpureus rice preparation: a placebo-controlled, double-blind clinical trial. Paper presented at: 39th Annual Conference on Cardiovascular Disease Epidemiology and Prevention, 1999; Orlando, FL.

380. Rippe J, Bonovich K, Colfer H. A multi-center, self-controlled study of Cholestin [TM] in subjects with elevated cholesterol. Paper presented at: 39th Annual Conference on Cardiovascular Disease Epidemiology and Prevention., 1999; Orlando, FL.

381. Wang J, Lu Z, Chi J. Multicenter clinical trial of the serum lipid-lowering effects of a Monascus purpureus (red yeast) rice preparation from traditional Chinese medicine. *Cur Ther Res.* 1997;58:964-978.

382. Pieper JA. Understanding niacin formulations. *Am J Manag Care.* 2002;8(12 Suppl):S308-314.

383. Tavintharan S, Kashyap ML. The benefits of niacin in atherosclerosis. *Curr Atheroscler Rep.* 2001;3(1):74-82.

384. O'Connor PJ, Rush WA, Trence DL. Relative effectiveness of niacin and lovastatin for treatment of dyslipidemias in a health maintenance organization. *J Fam Pract.* 1997;44(5):462-467.

385. Sakai T, Kamanna VS, Kashyap ML. Niacin, but not gemfibrozil, selectively increases LP-AI, a cardioprotective subfraction of HDL, in patients with low HDL cholesterol. *Arterioscler Thromb Vasc Biol.* 2001;21(11):1783-1789.

386. Ito MK. Niacin-based therapy for dyslipidemia: past evidence and future advances. *Am J Manag Care.* 2002;8(12 Suppl):S315-322.

387. Pan J, Lin M, Kesala RL, Van J, Charles MA. Niacin treatment of the atherogenic lipid profile and Lp(a) in diabetes. *Diabetes Obes Metab.* 2002;4(4):255-261.

388. McCarty MF. Inhibition of acetyl-CoA carboxylase by cystamine may mediate the hypotriglyceridemic activity of pantethine. *Med Hypotheses.* 2001;56(3):314-317.

389. Durak a A, Ozturk HS, Olcay E, Guven C. Effects of garlic extract supplementation on blood lipid and antioxidant parameters and atherosclerotic plaque formation process in cholesterol-fed rabbits. *J Herb Pharmcother.* 2002;2(2):19-32.

390. Saravanan G, Prakash J. Effect of garlic (Allium sativum) on lipid peroxidation in experimental myocardial infarction in rats. *J Ethnopharmacol.* 2004;94(1):155-158.

391. Orekhov AN, Grunwald J. Effects of garlic on atherosclerosis. *Nutrition.* 1997;13(7-8):656-663.

392. Campbell JH, Efendy JL, Smith NJ, Campbell GR. Molecular basis by which garlic suppresses atherosclerosis. *J Nutr.* 2001;131(3s):1006S-1009S.

393. Ho SE, Ide N, Lau BH. S-allyl cysteine reduces oxidant load in cells involved in the atherogenic process. *Phytomedicine.* 2001;8(1):39-46.

394. Jain AK, Vargas R, Gotzkowsky S, McMahon FG. Can garlic reduce levels of serum lipids? A controlled clinical study. *Am J Med.* 1993;94(6):632-635.

395. Lawson LD, Wang ZJ, Papadimitriou D. Allicin release under simulated gastrointestinal conditions from garlic powder tablets employed in clinical trials on serum cholesterol. *Planta Med.* 2001;67(1):13-18.

396. Mader FH. Treatment of hyperlipidaemia with garlic-powder tablets. Evidence from the German Association of General Practitioners' multicentric placebo-controlled double-blind study.

Arzneimittelforschung. 1990;40(10):1111-1116.

397. Urizar NL, Moore DD. GUGULIPID: a natural cholesterol-lowering agent. *Annu Rev Nutr.* 2003;23:303-313. Epub 2003 Feb 2026.

398. Singh RB, Niaz MA, Ghosh S. Hypolipidemic and antioxidant effects of Commiphora mukul as an adjunct to dietary therapy in patients with hypercholesterolemia. *Cardiovasc Drugs Ther.* 1994;8(4):659-664

399. Nityanand S, Srivastava JS, Asthana OP. Clinical trials with gugulipid. A new hypolipidaemic agent. *J Assoc Physicians India.* 1989;37(5):323-328.

400. Dalvi SS, Nayak VK, Pohujani SM, Desai NK, Kshirsagar NA, Gupta KC. Effect of gugulipid on bioavailability of diltiazem and propranolol. *J Assoc Physicians India.* 1994;42(6):454-455

401. Anderson JW, Gilinsky NH, Deakins DA, et al. Lipid responses of hypercholesterolemic men to oat-bran and wheat-bran intake. *Am J Clin Nutr.* 1991;54(4):678-683.

402. Whyte JL, McArthur R, Topping D, Nestel P. Oat bran lowers plasma cholesterol levels in mildly hypercholesterolemic men. *J Am Diet Assoc.* 1992;92(4):446-449.

403. Winblad I, Joensuu T, Korpela H. Effect of oat bran supplemented diet on hypercholesterolaemia. *Scand J Prim Health Care.* 1995;13(2):118-121.

404. Ajani UA, Ford ES, Mokdad AH. Dietary fiber and C-reactive protein: findings from national health and nutrition examination survey data. *J Nutr.* 2004;134(5):1181-1185.

405. King DE, Egan BM, Geesey ME. Relation of dietary fat and fiber to elevation of C-reactive protein. *Am J Cardiol.* 2003;92(11):1335-1339.

406. Liu S, Manson JE, Stampfer MJ, et al. Whole grain consumption and risk of ischemic stroke in women: A prospective study. *Jama.* 2000;284(12):1534-1540.

407. Ascherio A, Rimm EB, Hernan MA, et al. Intake of potassium, magnesium, calcium, and fiber and risk of stroke among US men. *Circulation.* 1998;98(12):1198-1204.

408. Bazzano LA, He J, Ogden LG, Loria CM, Whelton PK. Dietary fiber intake and reduced risk of coronary heart disease in US men and women: the National Health and Nutrition Examination Survey I Epidemiologic Follow-up Study. *Arch Intern Med.* 2003;163(16):1897-1904.

409. Wagenaar LJ, Voors AA, Buikema H, van Gilst WH. Angiotensin receptors in the cardiovascular system. *Can J Cardiol.* 2002;18(12):1331-1339.

410. Li YC, Kong J, Wei M, Chen ZF, Liu SQ, Cao LP. 1,25-Dihydroxyvitamin D(3) is a negative endocrine regulator of the renin-angiotensin system. *J Clin Invest.* 2002;110(2):229-238.

411. Li YC. Vitamin D regulation of the renin-angiotensin system. *J Cell Biochem.* 2003;88(2):327-331.

412. Hansen K, Nyman U, Smitt UW, et al. In vitro screening of traditional medicines for anti-hypertensive effect based on inhibition of the angiotensin converting enzyme (ACE). *J Ethnopharmacol.* 1995;48(1):43-51.

413. Lacaille D, Franck U, Wagner H. Search for potential angiotensin converting enzyme (ACE)-inhibitors from plants. *Phytomedicine.* 2001;8(1):47-52.

414. Czap K. *Alternative Medicine Review - Monographs.* Vol 1. Dover, Idaho: Thorne Research; 2002.

415. De Meyer GR, De Cleen DM, Cooper S, et al. Platelet phagocytosis and processing of beta-amyloid precursor protein as a mechanism of macrophage activation in atherosclerosis. *Circ Res.* 2002;90(11):1197-1204.

416. Ichii T, Koyama H, Tanaka S, et al. Thrombospondin-1 mediates smooth muscle cell proliferation induced by interaction with human platelets. *Arterioscler Thromb Vasc Biol.* 2002;22(8):1286-1292.

417. Nassar T, Sachais BS, Akkawi S, et al. Platelet factor 4 enhances the binding of oxidized low-density lipoprotein to vascular wall cells. *J Biol Chem.* 2003;278(8):6187-6193. Epub 2002 Dec 6103.

418. Smith PF, Maclennan K, Darlington CL. The neuroprotective properties of the Ginkgo biloba leaf: a review of the possible relationship to platelet-activating factor (PAF). *J Ethnopharmacol.* 1996;50(3):131-139.

419. Hostettler ME, Knapp PE, Carlson SL. Platelet-activating factor induces cell death in cultured astrocytes and oligodendrocytes: involvement of caspase-3. *Glia.* 2002;38(3):228-239.

420. Tselepis AD, John Chapman M. Inflammation, bioactive lipids and atherosclerosis: potential roles of a lipoprotein-associated phospholipase A2, platelet activating factor-acetylhydrolase. *Atheroscler Suppl.* 2002;3(4):57-68.

421. Zhou LJ, Song W, Zhu XZ, Chen ZL, Yin ML, Cheng XF. Protective effects of bilobalide on amyloid beta-peptide 25-35-induced PC12 cell cytotoxicity. *Acta Pharmacol Sin.* 2000;21(1):75-79.

422. Liu C, Qian G, Liu H. [Experimental study on suppressive effect of ginkgo extract on adhesion of vascular endothelial cell to monocyte induced by minimally modified low density lipoprotein]. *Zhongguo Zhong Xi Yi Jie He Za Zhi.* 2000;20(12):917-919.

423. Lin SJ, Yang TH, Chen YH, et al. Effects of Ginkgo biloba extract on the proliferation of vascular smooth muscle cells in vitro and on intimal thickening and interleukin-1beta expression after balloon injury in cholesterol-fed rabbits in vivo. *J Cell Biochem.* 2002;85(3):572-582.

424. Wei Z, Peng Q, Lau BH, Shah V. Ginkgo biloba inhibits hydrogen peroxide-induced activation of nuclear factor kappa B in vascular endothelial cells. *Gen Pharmacol.* 1999;33(5):369-375.

425. Unal I, Gursoy-Ozdemir Y, Bolay H, Soylemezoglu F, Saribas O, Dalkara T. Chronic daily administration of selegiline and EGb 761 increases brain's resistance to ischemia in mice. *Brain Res.* 2001;917(2):174-181.

426. Zhang WR, Hayashi T, Kitagawa H, et al. Protective effect of ginkgo extract on rat brain with transient middle cerebral artery occlusion. *Neurol Res.* 2000;22(5):517-521.

427. Sasaki Y, Noguchi T, Yamamoto E, et al. Effects of Ginkgo biloba extract (EGb 761) on cerebral thrombosis and blood pressure in stroke-prone spontaneously hypertensive rats. *Clin Exp Pharmacol Physiol.* 2002;29(11):963-967.

428. Defeudis FV. Bilobalide and neuroprotection. *Pharmacol Res.* 2002;46(6):565-568.

429. Kleijnen J, Knipschild P. The comprehensiveness of Medline and Embase computer searches. Searches for controlled trials of homoeopathy, ascorbic acid for common cold and ginkgo biloba for cerebral insufficiency and intermittent claudication. *Pharm Weekbl Sci.* 1992;14(5):316-320.

430. Hopfenmuller W. [Evidence for a therapeutic effect of Ginkgo biloba special extract. Meta-analysis of 11 clinical studies in patients with cerebrovascular insufficiency in old age]. *Arzneimittelforschung.* 1994;44(9):1005-1013.

431. Garg RK, Nag D, Agrawal A. A double blind placebo controlled trial of ginkgo biloba extract in acute cerebral ischaemia. *J Assoc Physicians India.* 1995;43(11):760-763.

432. See note 414 above.

433. Molnar P, Erdo SL. Vinpocetine is as potent as phenytoin to block voltage-gated Na+ channels in rat cortical neurons. *Eur J Pharmacol.* 1995;273(3):303-306.

434. Urenjak J, Obrenovitch TP. Neuroprotection–rationale for pharmacological modulation of Na(+)-channels. *Amino Acids.* 1998;14(1-3):151-158.

435. Bonoczk P, Panczel G, Nagy Z. Vinpocetine increases cerebral blood flow and oxygenation in stroke patients: a near infrared spectroscopy and transcranial Doppler study. *Eur J Ultrasound.* 2002;15(1-2):85-91.

436. Feigin VL, Doronin BM, Popova TF, Gribatcheva EV, Tchervov DV. Vinpocetine treatment in acute ischaemic stroke: a pilot single-blind randomized clinical trial. *Eur J Neurol.* 2001;8(1):81-85.

437. Vas A, Gulyas B, Szabo Z, et al. Clinical and non-clinical investigations using positron emission tomography, near infrared spectroscopy and transcranial Doppler methods on the neuroprotective drug vinpocetine: a summary of evidences. *J Neurol Sci.* 2002;203-204:259-262.

438. Hagiwara M, Endo T, Hidaka H. [Effect of vinpocetine (TCV-3B), a vasodilator agent, on cyclic nucleotide metabolism]. *Nippon Yakurigaku Zasshi.* 1982;80(4):317-323.

439. Hagiwara M, Endo T, Hidaka H. Effects of vinpocetine on cyclic nucleotide metabolism in vascular smooth muscle. *Biochem Pharmacol.* 1984;33(3):453-457.

440. Yasui M, Yano I, Ota K, Oshima A. Preventive effect of vinpocetine on calcifications: atherosclerosis in experimental rabbits. *Acta Neurol Scand.* 1989;79(3):239-242.

441. Yasui M, Yano I, Ota K, Oshima A. [Contents of calcium, phosphorus and aluminum in central nervous system, liver and kidney of rabbits with experimental atherosclerosis–scavenger effects of vinpocetine on the deposition of elements]. *No To Shinkei.* 1990;42(4):325-331.

442. Yasui M, Yano I, Ota K, Oshima A. Calcium, phosphorus and aluminium concentrations in the central nervous system, liver and kidney of rabbits with experimental atherosclerosis: preventive effects of vinpocetine on the deposition of these elements. *J Int Med Res.* 1990;18(2):142-152.

443. Majors AK, Sengupta S, Jacobsen DW, Pyeritz RE. Upregulation of smooth muscle cell collagen production by homocysteine-insight into the pathogenesis of homocystinuria. *Mol Genet Metab.*

2002;76(2):92-99.

444. Weiss N, Keller C, Hoffmann U, Loscalzo J. Endothelial dysfunction and atherothrombosis in mild hyperhomocysteinemia. *Vasc Med.* 2002;7(3):227-239.

445. Signorello MG, Pascale R, Leoncini G. Effect of homocysteine on arachidonic acid release in human platelets. *Eur J Clin Invest.* 2002;32(4):279-284.

446. Willinek WA, Ludwig M, Lennarz M, Holler T, Stumpe KO. High-normal serum homocysteine concentrations are associated with an increased risk of early atherosclerotic carotid artery wall lesions in healthy subjects. *J Hypertens.* 2000;18(4):425-430.

447. Sasaki T, Watanabe M, Nagai Y, et al. Association of plasma homocysteine concentration with atherosclerotic carotid plaques and lacunar infarction. *Stroke.* 2002;33(6):1493-1496.

448. Apeland T, Mansoor MA, Pentieva K, McNulty H, Seljeflot I, Strandjord RE. The effect of B-vitamins on hyperhomocysteinemia in patients on antiepileptic drugs. *Epilepsy Res.* 2002;51(3):237-247.

449. Rogers JD, Sanchez-Saffon A, Frol AB, Diaz-Arrastia R. Elevated plasma homocysteine levels in patients treated with levodopa: association with vascular disease. *Arch Neurol.* 2003;60(1):59-64.

450. Verhoef P, Pasman WJ, Van Vliet T, Urgert R, Katan MB. Contribution of caffeine to the homocysteine-raising effect of coffee: a randomized controlled trial in humans. *Am J Clin Nutr.* 2002;76(6):1244-1248.

451. Hirsch S, Pia De la Maza M, Yanez P, et al. Hyperhomocysteinemia and endothelial function in young subjects: effects of vitamin supplementation. *Clin Cardiol.* 2002;25(11):495-501.

452. Toole JF. Vitamin intervention for stroke prevention. *J Neurol Sci.* 2002;203-204:121-124.

453. Tanne D, Medalie JH, Goldbourt U. Body fat distribution and long-term risk of stroke mortality. *Stroke.* 2005;36(5):1021-1025. Epub 2005 Mar 1031.

454. Walker SP, Rimm EB, Ascherio A, Kawachi I, Stampfer MJ, Willett WC. Body size and fat distribution as predictors of stroke among US men. *Am J Epidemiol.* 1996;144(12):1143-1150.

455. Ernst E. Regular exercise reduces fibrinogen levels: a review of longitudinal studies. *Br J Sports Med.* 1993;27(3):175-176.

456. Goldhammer E, Tanchilevitch A, Maor I, Beniamini Y, Rosenschein U, Sagiv M. Exercise training modulates cytokines activity in coronary heart disease patients. *Int J Cardiol.* 2005;100(1):93-99.

457. Petersen AM, Pedersen BK. The anti-inflammatory effect of exercise. *J Appl Physiol.* 2005;98(4):1154-1162.

458. Wendel-Vos GC, Schuit AJ, Feskens EJ, et al. Physical activity and stroke. A meta-analysis of observational data. *Int J Epidemiol.* 2004;33(4):787-798. Epub 2004 May 2027.

459. Lee CD, Folsom AR, Blair SN. Physical activity and stroke risk: a meta-analysis. *Stroke.* 2003;34(10):2475-2481. Epub 2003 Sep 2418.

460. Ellekjaer H, Holmen J, Ellekjaer E, Vatten L. Physical activity and stroke mortality in women. Ten-year follow-up of the Nord-Trondelag health survey, 1984-1986. *Stroke.* 2000;31(1):14-18.

461. Bhathena SJ, Ali AA, Mohamed AI, Hansen CT, Velasquez MT. Differential effects of dietary flaxseed protein and soy protein on plasma triglyceride and uric acid levels in animal models. *J Nutr Biochem.* 2002;13(11):684-689.

462. Lichtenstein AH, Jalbert SM, Adlercreutz H, et al. Lipoprotein response to diets high in soy or animal protein with and without isoflavones in moderately hypercholesterolemic subjects. *Arterioscler Thromb Vasc Biol.* 2002;22(11):1852-1858.

463. Hu FB, Bronner L, Willett WC, et al. Fish and omega-3 fatty acid intake and risk of coronary heart disease in women. *Jama.* 2002;287(14):1815-1821.

464. von Schacky C, Baumann K, Angerer P. The effect of n-3 fatty acids on coronary atherosclerosis: results from SCIMO, an angiographic study, background and implications. *Lipids.* 2001;36(Suppl):S99-102.

465. Thies F, Garry JM, Yaqoob P, et al. Association of n-3 polyunsaturated fatty acids with stability of atherosclerotic plaques: a randomised controlled trial. *Lancet.* 2003;361(9356):477-485.

466. Maier JA. Low magnesium and atherosclerosis: an evidence-based link. *Mol Aspects Med.* 2003;24(1-3):137-146.

467. See Note 407 above.

468. Landmark K. [Hypokalemia can accelerate the development of cerebrovascular and cardiovascular disease]. *Tidsskr Nor Laegeforen.* 2002;122(5):499-501.

469. Stampfli S. The antioxidative and anti-inflammatory properties of PADMA 28. *Schweiz. Zschr. GanzheitsMedzin.* 2001;13:242-245.

470. Winther K. Padma 28, a botanical compound decreases the oxidative burst reaction of monocytes and improves fibrinolysis in patients with stable intermittent claudication. *Fibrinolysis.* 1994;8(2):47-49.

471. Drabaek H, Mehlsen J, Himmelstrup H, Winther K. A botanical compound, Padma 28, increases walking distance in stable intermittent claudication. *Angiology*. 1993;44(11):863-867.

472. Wojcicki J, Samochowiec L. Controlled double-blind study of Padma 28 in Angina Pectoris. *Herba Polonica*. 1986;32:107-114.

473. Gladysz A. Influence of Padma 28 on Patients with Chronic Active Hepatitis Type B. *Phytotherapy Research*. 1993;7:244-247.

474. Brzosko WJ. Influence of PADMA 28 and thymus extract on clinical and laboratory parameters of children with juvenile chronic arthritis. *Int Journal of Immunotherapy*. 1991;7(3):143-147.

475. Jankowski A. Treatment with PADMA 28 of children with recurrent infections of the respiratory tract. *Therapiewoche Schweiz*. 1986;2(1):25-32.

476. Korwin-Piotrowska T. Experience of Padma 28 in Multiple Sclerosis. *Phytotherapy Research*. 1991;6:133-136.

477. Brunner-La Rocca HP, Schindler R, Schlumpf M, Saller R, Suter M. Effects of the Tibetan herbal preparation PADMA 28 on blood lipids and lipid oxidisability in subjects with mild hypercholesterolaemia. *Vasa*. 2005;34(1):11-17.

478. Barak V, Kalickman I, Halperin T, Birkenfeld S, Ginsburg I. PADMA-28, a Tibetan herbal preparation is an inhibitor of inflammatory cytokine production. *Eur Cytokine Netw*. 2004;15(3):203-209.

479. Moskowitz MA. The neurobiology of vascular head pain. *Ann Neurol*. 1984 Aug;16(2):157-68.

480. Moskowitz MA. Basic mechanisms in vascular headaches. *Neurol Clinc*. 1990 Nov;8(4):801-15.

481. Ahmed M, et al. Capsaicin effects on substance P and CRGP in rat adjuvant arthritis. *Regul Pept*. 1995 Jan 5;55(1):85-102.

482. Sarchielli P, et al. Chemokine levels in the jugular venous blood of migraine without aura patients during attacks. *Headache*. 2004 Nov-Dec;44(10):961-8.

483. Bolay H, et al. Intrinsic brain activity triggers trigeminal meningeal afferents in a migraine model. *Nat Med*. 2002 Feb;8(2):136-42.

484. Sanchez-del-Rio M and Reuter U. Migraine aura: new information on underlying mechanisms. *Curr Opin Neurol*. 2004 Jun;17(3):289-93.

485. Knight YE and Goadsby PJ. The periaqueductal grey matter modulates trigeminovascular input; a role in migraine? *Neuroscience.* 2001;106(4):793-800.

486. Welch KM, et al. Periaqueductal gray matter dysfunction in migraine: cause or the burden of illness? *Headache.* 2001 Jul-Aug;41(7):629-37.

487. Ashcroft FM From molecule to malady. *Nature.* 2006 Mar 23;440(7083):440.

488. Barrett CF, Cao YQ, Tsien RW. Gating deficiency in a familial hemiplegic migraine type 1 mutant P/Q-type calcium channel. *J Biol Chem.* 2005 Jun 24;280(25):24064-71. Epub 2005 Mar 28.

489. Knight YE, Bartsch T, Kaube H, Goadsby PJ. P/Q-type calcium-channel blockade in the periqaqueductal gray facilitates trigeminal nociception: a functional genetic link for migraine? *J Neurosci.* 2002 Mar 1;22(5):RC213.

490. Gallai V, Sarchielli P, Morucci P, Abbritti G. Red blood cell magnesium levels in migraine patients. *Cephalagia.* 1993 Apr;13(2):94-81; discussion 73.

491. Schenen J, Sienard-Gainko J, Lenaerts M. Bloog magnesium levels in migraine. *Cephalalgia.* 1991 May;11(2):97-9.

492. Sarchielli P, Coata G, Firenze C, Morucci P, Abbritti G, Gallai V. Serum and salivary magnesium levels ion migraine and tension-type headache. Results in a group of adult patients. *Cephalagia.* 1992 Feb;12(1):21-7.

493. MauskopA, Altura BM. Role of magnesium in the pathogenesis and treatment of migraines. *Clin Neurosci.* 1998; 5(1):24-7.

494. Voets T, Janssens A, Prenen J, Droohmans G, Nilius B. Mg++-dependent gating and strong inward rectification of the cation channel TRPV6. *J Gen Physiol.* 2003 Mar;121(3):245-60.

495. McCarty MF. Complementary vascular-protective actions of magnesium and taurine: a rationale for magnesium taurate. *Med Hypotheses.* 1996 Feb;46(2):89-100.

496. Matsushima Y, et al. Effects of taurine on serum cholesterol levels and development of atherosclerosis in spontaneously hyperlipidaemic mice. *Clin Exp Pharmacol Physiol.* 2003 Apr;30(4):295-9.

497. Miglis M, Wilder D, Reid T, Bakaltcheva I. Effect of taurine on platelets and the plasma coagulation system. *Platelets.* 2002 Feb;13(1):5-10.

498. Chen WQ, et al. Role of taurine in regulation of intracellular calcium level and neuroprotective function in cultured neurons. *J Neurosci Res*. 2001 Nov 15;66(4):612-9.

499. Wu H, Jin Y, Wei J, Jin H, Sha D, Wu JY. Mode of action of taurine as a neuroprotector. *Brain Res*. 2005 Mar 21;1038(2):123-31.

500. Louzada PR, et al. Taurine prevents the neurotoxicity of beta-amyloid and glutamate receptor agonists: activation of GABA receptors and possible implications for Alzheimer's disease and other neurological disorders. *FASEB J*. 2004 Mar;18(3):511-8.

501. Koga Y and Nataliya P. Migrine headache and mitochondrial DNA abnormality. *Nippon Rinsho*. 2005 Oct;63(10):1710-6.

502. Okada H, Araga S, Takeshima T, Nakashima K. Plasma lactic acid and pyruvic acid levels in migraine and tension-type headache. *Headache*. 1998 Jan;38(1):39-42.

503. Welch KM, Levine SR, D'Andrea G, Schultz LR, Helpern JA. Preliminary observations on brain energy metabolism in migraine studied by in-vivo phosphorus NMR spectroscopy. *Neurology*. 1989 Apr;39(4):538-41.

504. Barbiroli, et al. Abnormal brain and muscle energy metabolism shown by 31P magneic resonance spectroscopy in patients affected by migraine with aura. *Neurology*. 1992 Jun;42(6):1209-14.

505. Montagna P, et al. 31P-magnetic resonance spectroscopy in migraine without aura. *Neurology*. 1994 Apr;44(4):666-9.

506. Lodi R, et al. Deficient energy metabolism is associated with low free magnesium in the brain of patients with migraine and cluster headaches. *Brain Re Bull*. 2001 Mar 1;54(4):437-41.

507. Buresh Ia, Koroleva VI, Gorelova AN. Leao's spreading depression: synaptic regulation of a diffuse self-oscillating process in the etral nervous system. *Neirofiziologiia*. 1984;16(5): 702-16.

508. Rozen TD. Open label trial of coenzyme Q10 as a migraine preventive. *Cephalalgia*. 2002 Mar;22(2):137-41.

509. Sandor PS. Efficacy of coenzyme Q10 in migraine prophylaxis: a randomized controlled trial. *Neurology*. 2005 Feb 22;64(4):713-5.

510. Schoene J, Jacquy J, Lenaerts M. Effective of high-dose riboflavin in migraine prophylaxis. A randomized controlled trial. *Neurolog*. 1998 Feb;50(2):466-70.

511. Boehnke C, et al. High-dose riboflavin treatment is efficacious in migraine prophylaxis: an open study in a tertiary care centre. *Eur J Neurol*. 2004 Jul;11(7):475-7.

512. Liu J, Killilea DW, Ames BN. Age-associated mitochondrial oxidative decay: improvement of carnitine acetyltransferase substrate-binding affinity and activity in brain by feeding old rats acetyl-L-carnitine and/or R-alpha-lipoic acid. *Proc Natl Acad Sci U.S.A.* 2002 Feb 19;99(4):1876-81.

513. Jiankang Liu, et al. Delaying brain mitochondrial decay and aging with mitochondrial antioxidants and metabolites. *Ann N Y Acad Sci.* 2002 Apr;959:133-66.

514. Makheja AN, Bailey JM. A platelet phospholipase inhibitor from the medicinal herb feverfew (Tanacetum parthenium). *Prostaglandins Leukot Med.* 1982 Jun;8(6):653-60.

515. Kwok BH, et al. The anti-inflammatory natural product parthenolide from the medicinal herb Feverfew directly binds to and inhibits IkappaB kinase. *Chem Biol.* 2001 Aug;8(8):759-66.

516. Reuter U, et al. Nuclear factor-kappaB as a molecular target for migraine therapy. *Ann Neurol.* 2002 Apr;51(4):507-16.

517. Tassorelli C, et al. Parthenolide is the component of tanacetum parthenium that inhibits nitroglycerin-induced Fos activation: studies in an animal model of migraine. *Cephalalgia.* 2005 Aug;25(8):612-21.

518. Pittler MH, Ernst E. Feverfew for preventing migraine. *Cochrane Database Syst Rev.* 2004;(1):CD002286.

519. Efficacy and safety of 6.25mg T.I.D. feverfew CO2-extract (MIG-99) in migraine prevention-a randomized, double-blind, multicentre, placebo-controlled study. *Cephalalgia.* 2005 Nov;25(11):1031-41.

520. Johnson ES, et al. Efficacy of feverfew as prophylactic treatment of migraine. *Br Med J (Clin Res Ed).* 1985 Aug 31;291(6495):596-73.

521. Murphy JJ, et al. Randomized double-blind placebo-controlled trial of feverfew in migraine prevention. *Lancet.* 1988 Jul 23;2(8604):189-92.

522. Khan SI, et al. Transport of parthenolide across human intestinal cells (Caca-2). *Planta Med.* 2003 Nov;69(11):1009-12.

523. Heptinstall S, et al. Parthenolide content and bioactivity of feverfew (Tanacetum parthenum (L.) Schultz-Bip.). Estimation of commercial and authenticated feverfew products. *J Pharm Pharmacol.* 1992 May;44(5):391-5.

524. Fiebich BL, et al. Petasites hybridus extracts in vitro inhibit COX-2 and PGE2 release by direct interaction with the enzyme and by preventing p42/44 MAP kinase activation in rat primary microglial cells. *Planta Med.* 2005 Jan;71(1):12-9.

525. LaPointe MC, Isenovic E. Interleukin-1beta regulation of inducible nitric oxide synthase and cyclooxygenase-2 involves the p42/44 and p38 MAPK signaling pathway in cardiac myocytes. *Hypertension.* 1999 Jan;33(1 Pt 2):276-82.

526. Wang, et al. Calcium-antagonizing activity of S-petasin, a hypotensive sesquiterpene from Petasites formosanus, on inotropic and chronotropic responses in isolated rat atria and cardiac myocytes. *Naunyn Schmiedebergs Arch Pharmacol.* 2004 Mar;369(3):322-9. Epub 2004 Feb 4.

527. Ko WC, et al. Mechanisms of relaxant action of S-petasin and S-isopetasin, sesquiterpenes of Petasites formosanus, in isolated guinea pig traches. *Planta Med.* 2001 Apr;67(3):224-9.

528. Wu Sn, et al. The mechanism of inhibitory actions of S-petasin, a sesquiterpene of Petasites formosanus, on L-tupe calcium current in NG108-15 neuronal cells. *Planta Med.* 2003 Feb;69(2):118-24.

529. Diener HC, et al. The first placebo-controlled trial of a special butterbur root extract for the prevention of migraine: reanalysis of efficacy criteria. *Eur Neurol.* 2004;51(2):89-97. Epub 2004 Jan 26.

530. Grossman W and Schmidramsl H. An extract of Petasites hybridus is effective ion the prophylaxis of migraine. *Altern Med Rev.* 2001 Jun;6(3):303-10.

531. Lipton RB, et al. Petasites hybridus root (Butterbur) is an effective preventive treatment for migraine. *Neurology.* 2004 Dec 28:63(12):2240-4.

532. Ropper, Allan and Brown, Robert. *Adams and Victor's Principles of Neurology.* Eighth Edition. McGraw Hill. 2005. page 271.

533. Kim WJ, et al. The prognosis for control of seizures with medications in patients with MRI evidence for mesial temporal sclerosis. *Epilepsia.* 1999 Mar;40(3):290-3.

534. Ropper, Allan and Brown, Robert. *Adams and Victor's Principles of Neurology.* Eighth Edition. McGraw Hill. 2005. page 282

535. Armijo JA. Ion channels and epilepsy. *Curr Pharm Des.* 2005;11(15):1975-2003.

536. Loscher W. Basic pharmacology of valproate: a review after 35 years of clinical use for the treatment of epilepsy. *CNS Drugs.* 2002;16(10):669-94.

537. Campo-Soria C, et al. Mechanism of action of benzodiazepines on GABAA receptors. *Br J Pharmacol.* 2006 Aug;148(7):984-90. Epub 2006 Jun 19.

538. Wood JH, et al. Low cerebrospinal fluid gamma-aminobutyric acid content in seizure patients. *Neurology.* 1979 Sep;29(9 Pt 1):1203-8.

539. Yamamoto M, et al. GABA levels in cerebrospinal fluid of patients with epilepsy. *Folia Psychiatr Neurol Jpn.* 1985;39(4):515-9.

540. Petroff OA, et al. Low brain GABA level is associated with poor seizure control. *Ann Neurol.* 1996 Dec;40(6):908-11.

541. Thwaites Dt, et al. Gamma-aminobutryric acid (GABA) transport across human intestinal epithelial (Caco-2) cell monolayers. *Br J Pharmacol.* 2000 Feb;129(3):457-64.

542. Zhang Y and Liu GQ. Sodium and chloride-dependent high and low-affinity uptakes of GABA by brain capillary endothelial cells. *Brain Res.* 1999 Oct 12;808(1):1-7.

543. Zhang Y and Liu G. A novel method to determine the localization of high and low-affinity GABA transporters to the luminal and antiluminal membranes of brain capillary endothelial cells. *Brain Res Protoc.* 1999 Dec;4(3):288-94..

544. Takanaga H, et al. GAT2/BGT-1 as a system responsible for the transport of gamma-aminobutyric at the mouse blood-brain barrier. *J cereb Blood Flow Metab.* 2001 Oct;21(10):1232-9.

545. Vignolo L, et al. Accumulation of labeled gamma-aminobutyric acid into rat brain and brain synaptosomes after i.p. injection. *Neurochem Res.* 1992 Feb;17(2):193-9.

546. Benassi, et al. Evaluation of the mechanism by which gamma-amino-butyric acid in association with phosphatidylserine exerts an antiepileptic effect in the rat. *Neurochem Res.* 1992 Dec;17(12):1229-33.

547. Thwaites DT, et al. Gamma-Aminobutyric acid (GABA) transport across human intestinal epithelial (Caco-2) cell monolayers. *Br J Pharmacol.* 2000 Feb;120(3):457-64.

548. Streeter JG and Thompson JF. In vivo and in vitro studies on gamma-aminobutyric acid metabolism with the radish plant (Raphanus sativus L.) *Plant Physiol.* (1972) 49, 579-584.

549. Riedel G, et al. Glutamate receptor function in learning and memory. *Behav Brain Res.* 2003 Mar 18;140(1-2):1-47.

550. Shulgins GI. On neurotransmitter mechanisms of reinforcement and internal inhibition. *Pavlov J Biol Sci.* 1986 Oct-Dec;21(4):129-40.

551. Ziablintseva EA. The effect of GABA derivative phenibut on defensive conditioning and internal inhibition. *Zh Vyesh Nerv Deiat Im I P Pavlova.* 2006 Mar-Apr;56(2):236-41.

552. Patel AB, et al. The contribution of GABA to glutamate/glutamine cycling and energy metabolism in the rat cortex in vivo. *Proc Natl Acad Sci USA*. 2005 Apr 12;102(15):5588-93. Epub 2005 Apr 4.

553. Meldrum BS, et al. Glutamate receptors and transporters in genetic and acquired models of epilepsy. *Epilepsy Res.* 1999 Sep;36(2-3):189-204.

554. Chen WQ, et al. Role of taurine in regulation of intracellular calcium level and neuroprotective function in cultured neurons. *J Neurosci Res.* 2001 Nov 15:66(4):612-9.

555. Wu H, et al. Mode of action of taurine as a neuroprotector. *Brain Res.* 2005 Mar 21;1038(2):123-31.

556. Sulaiman SA, et al. Kinetic studies on the inhibition of GABA-T by gamma-vinyl GABA and taurine. *J Enzyme Inhibit Med Chem.* 2003 Aug;18(4):297-301.

557. Rainesalo S, et al. Plasma and cerebrospinal fluid amino acids in epileptic patients. *Neurochem Res.* 2004 Jan;29(1):319-24.

558. Dahlin M, et al. The ketogenic diet influences the levels of excitatory and inhibitory amino acids in the CSF in children with refractory epilepsy. *Epilepsy Res.* 2005 May;64(3):115-25.

559. El Idrissi A, et al. Prevention of epileptic seizures by taurine. *Adv Exp Med Biol.* 2003;426:515-25.

560. Konig P, et al. Orally-administered taurine in therapy-resistant epilepsy (author's transl) (Article in German). *Wien Klin Wochenschr.* 1977 Feb 10;89(4):111-3.

561. Marchesi GF, et al. Therapeutic effects of taurine in epilepsy; a clinical and polyphysiographic study (author's transl) (Article in Italian). *Riv Patol Nerv Ment.* 1975 May-June;96(3):166-84.

562. Geggel HS, et al. Nutritional requirement for taurine in patients receiving long-term parenteral nutrition. *N Engl J Med.* 1985 Jan 17;312(3):142-6.

563. Kang YS, et al. Regulation of taurine transport at the blood-brain barrier by tumor necrosis factor-alpha, taurine and hypertonicity. *J Neurochem.* 2002 Dec;83(5):1188-95.

564. Stummer W, et al. Blood-brain barrier taurine transport during osmotic stress and in focal cerebral ischemia. *J Cereb Blood Flow Metab.* 1995 Sep;15(5):1852-9.

565. Oladipo OO, et al. Plasma magnesium in adult Nigerian patients with epilepsy. *Niger Postgrad Med J.* 2003 Dec;10(4):234-7.

566. Sood AK, et al. Serum, CSF, RBC and urinary levels of magnesium and calcium in idiopathic generalized tonic clonic seizures. *Indian J Med Res.* 1993 Jun;98:152-4.

567. Senga I, et al. Plasma and cerebrospinal fluid concentrations of magnesium in epileptic children. *J Neurol Sci.* 1985 Jan;67(1):29-34.

568. Dharnidharka VR and Carney PR Isolated idiopathic hypomagnesemia presenting as aphasia and seizures. *Pediatr Neurol.* 2005 Jul;33(1):61-5.

569. Weisleder P, et al. Hypomagnesemic seizures; case report and presumed pathophysiology. *J Child Neurol.* 2002 Jan;17(1);59-61.

570. Lazarini CA, Vassilieff I Does magnesium chloride modify aldrin-induced neurotoxicity in rats? *Vet Hum Toxicol.* 1998 Oct;40(5):257-9.

571. Cotton DB, et al. Central anticonvulsant effects of magnesium sulfate on N-methyl-D-aspartate-induced seizures. *Am J Obstet Gynecol.* 1993 Mar;168(3 Pt 1):974-8.

572. Magnesium is more efficacious than phenytoin in reducing N-methyl-D-aspartate seizures in rats. *Am J Obstet Gynecol.* 1994 Oct;171(4):999-1002.

573. Peredery O and Persinger MA Herbal treatment following post-seizure induction by lithium pilocarpine: Scutellaria lateriflora (Skullcap), Gelsmium sempervierns (Gelsmium) and Datura stramomium (Jimson weed) may prevent development of spontaneous seizures. *Phytother Res.* 2004 Sep;18(9):700-5.

574. Kumar V. Potential medicinal plants for CNS disorders: an overview. *Phytother Res.* 2006 Dec;20(12):1023-35.

575. Holcomb LA, et al. Bacopa monniera extract reduces amyloid levels in PSAPP mice. *J Alzheimer's Dis.* 2006 Aug;9(3):243-51.

576. Bhattacharya SK, et al. Antioxidant activity of Bacopa monniera in rat frontal cortex, striatum and hippocampus. *Phytother Res.* 2000 May;14(3):174-9.

577. Rai D, et al. Adaptogenic effect of Bacopa monniera (Brahmi). *Pharmacol Biochem Behav.* 2003 Jul;75(4):823-30.

578. Chowdhuri DK, et al. Antistress effects of bacosides of Bacopa monnieri: modulation of Hep70 expression, superoxide dismutase and cytochrome P450 activity in rat brain. *Phytother Res.* 2002 Nov;16(7):639-45.

579. Russo A, et al. Nitric oxide-related toxicity in cultured astrocytes: effect of Bacopa monniera. *Life Sci.* 2003 Aug 8;73(12):1517-26.

580. Russo A, et al. Free radical scavenging capacity and protective effect of Bacopa monniera L. on DNA damage. *Phytother Res.* 2003 Sep;17(8):870-5.

581. Stough C, et al. the chronic effects of an extract of Bacopa monniera (Brahmi) on cognitive function in healthy human subjects. *Psychopharmacology (Berl).* 2001 Aug;156(4):381-4.

582. Achliya GS, et al. Evaluation of sedative and anticonvulsant activities of Unmadnashak Ghrita. *J Ethnopharmacol.* 2004 Sep;94(1):77-83.

583. Vohora D, et al. Protection from phenytoin-induced cognitive deficit by Bacopa monniera, a reputed Indian nootropic plant. *J Ethnopharmacol.* 2000 Aug;71(3):383-90.

584. Mukherjee GD and Dey CD Clinical trial on Brahmi. I. *J Exp Med Sci.* 1966 Jun-Sep;10(1):5-11.

585. Santos MS, et al. Synaptosomal GABA release as influenced by valerian root extract–involvement of the GABA carrier. *Arch Inr Pharmacodyn Ther.* 1994 Mar-Apr;327(2):220-31.

586. Cavados C, et al. In vitro study on the interaction of Valerian officianalis L. extract and their amino acids on GABAA receptor in rat brain. *Arzneimittelforschung.* 1995 Jul;45(7):753-5.

587. Komori T, et al. The sleep-enhancing effect of valerian inhalation and sleep-shortening effect of lemon inhalation. *Chem Senses.* 2006 Oct;31(8):731-7.Epub 2006 Jul 20.

588. Dunaev VV, et al. Biological activity of the sum of the valepotriates isolated from Valeriana alliariifolia (Article in Russian). *Farmakol Toksikol.* 1987 Nov-Dec;50(6):33-7.

589. Sugaya A, et al. Inhibitory effect of peony root extract on pentylenetetrazol-induced EEG power spectrum changes and extracellular calcium concentration changes in rat cerebral cortex. *J Ethnopharmacol.* 1991 May-Jun;33(1-2).

590. Sunaga K, et al. Molecular mechanisms of preventative effect of peony root extract on neuron damage. *J Herb Pharmacother.* 2004;4(1):9-20.

591. Sugaya E, et al. Inhibitory effects of peony root extract on the large conductance calcium-activated potassium current essential in production of bursting activity. *J Herb Pharmacother.* 2006;6(2):65-77.

592. Dai Q, et al. Fruit and vegetable juices and Alzheimer's disease: the Kames project. *Am J Med.* 2006 Sep;119(9):791.

593. Zivadinov R, et al. HLA-DRB1*1501, -DQB*0301, -DQB1*0302, -DQB1*0602 and -DQB1*0603 Alleles are associated with more severe disease outcome on MRI in patients with multiple sclerosis. *Int. Rev. Neurobiol.* 2007;79:521-35.

594. Sidoti A, et al. Glyoxalase I A111E, paraoxonase 1 Q192R and L55M polymorphisms; susceptibility factors of multiple sclerosis? *Mult. Scler.* 2007m May;13(4):446-53.

595. Almeras L, et al. Developmental vitamin D deficiency alters brain protein expression in the adult rat: implications for neuropsychiatric disorders. *Proteomics.* 2007 Mar;7(5):769-80.

596. D, et al. Developmental vitamin D deficiency alters the expression of genes encoding mitochondrial, cytoskeletal and synaptic proteins in the adult rat brain. J Steroid Biochem. *Mol. Biol.* 2007 Mar;103(3-5):538-45. Epub 2006 Dec 23.

597. DeLuca GC, et al. The contribution of demyelination to axonal loss in multiple sclerosis. *Brain.* 2006 Jun;129 (Pt 6):1507-16. Epub 2006 Apr 5.

598. Bjartnar C, et al. Axonal loss in the pathology of MS: consequences for understanding the progressive phase of the disease. *J Neurol Sci.* 2003 Feb 15;206(2):165-71.

599. Andrews HE, et al. Mitochondrial dysfunction plays a key role in progressive axonal loss in multiple sclerosis. *Med. Hypothesis.* 2005;64(4):669-77.

600. Kalman B and Leist TP. A mitochondrial component of neurodegeneration in multiple sclerosis. *Neuromolecular Med.* 2003;3(3):147-58.

601. Moscarello MA, et al. The role of citrullinated proteins suggest a novel mechanism in the pathogenesis of multiple sclerosis. *Neurochem Res.* 2007 Feb; 32(2):251-6. Epub 2006 Sep 22.

602. Mastronardi FG, et al. Peptidyl argininedeiminase 2 CpG island in multiple sclerosis white matter is hypomethylated. *J Neurosci Res.* 2007 Apr 27; (Epub ahead of print).

603. Qin W, et al. Resveratrol induced DNA methylation in ER+ breast cancer. *Proc Amer Assoc Cancer Res.* Volume 46. 2005.

Index